WORKING WITH MEN
IN THE
HUMAN SERVICES

Edited by Bob Pease and Peter Camilleri

R Routledge
Taylor & Francis Group

LONDON AND NEW YORK

First published 2001 by Allen & Unwin

Published 2020 by Routledge
2 Park Square, Milton Park, Abingdon, Oxon OX14 4RN
605 Third Avenue, New York, NY 10017

Routledge is an imprint of the Taylor & Francis Group, an informa business

National Library of Australia
Cataloguing-in-Publication entry:

Working with men in the human services.

Bibliography.
Includes index.
ISBN 1 86508 480 8.

1. Masculinity. 2. Social service. 3. Men – Political aspects. I. Pease, Bob. II. Camilleri, Peter James.

305.31

Set in 10.5/12 pt Bembo by DOCUPRO, Sydney

ISBN-13: 9781865084800 (pbk)

Contents

Contributors

Graham Atkinson coordinates the Indigenous Studies elective in the School of Social Work at the University of Melbourne. He is a member of the Victorian Koori community and a member of the Yorta Yorta and Dja Dja Wuurrung clans. He has worked in Indigenous affairs for over 25 years and holds Bachelor of Arts and Social Work degrees from the University of Melbourne and an MBA from RMIT University.

Peter Camilleri is Associate Professor and Head of the School of Social Work at the Australian Catholic University in Canberra, where he is also Rector of the Signadou Campus. He has worked as a social worker in Tasmania, the Northern Territory and England and has been involved in the education of social workers for the past twelve years. He is President of the Australian Association of Social Work and Welfare Education and is the author of *(Re)Constructing Social Work* (Avebury 1996).

Mark Furlong is currently a lecturer in the Department of Social Work and Social Policy, Faculty of Health Services, La Trobe University where he has worked since mid-1995. Prior to commencing at La Trobe, Mark had undertaken direct practice roles for almost twenty years with a particular emphasis on work with families in mental health, disability and child protection. He has published broadly in psychiatric, family therapy, psychotherapeutic, social work and primary health journals.

Steve Golding has worked as a social worker in the South Australian health system for over fourteen years. He is currently Allied Health Coordinator in the Rural Health Training Unit. Steve has a small private practice and is a member of the Steering Committee developing a state-wide men's health and wellbeing policy in South Australia.

Mark Griffiths works at Anglicare (Victoria) as a Group Conference Convenor for the Juvenile Justice Conferencing Program. He has twenty years' experience in youth welfare and corrections and is currently undertaking postgraduate study on the topic of spirituality and social work practice.

Rob Hall has been working with men who abuse women since 1982. He is one of the founding members of the Domestic Violence Service and has worked with men, fathers and adolescent boys in relation to their violence. He has joined with other men and women to establish an independent counselling service—Nada. He is also currently working in a government service which assists adolescents and young men who have been sexually abused to adopt lives based on respect and care for others.

Mary Hood has practised social work mainly in the field of child and family welfare. This has involved work in disability services, statutory child protection, family therapy, residential care, specialist child abuse assessment and treatment and forensic work. In 1997 she completed a Doctorate in Social Science on the changing construction of child abuse over time and how this influenced professionals in direct interventions with children and families. She has published widely on this and related topics.

Peter Humprhies is a Manager of Social Work Services in the National Support Office of Centrelink in Canberra. He is a social worker with twenty years' experience in Education, Rehabilitation and Mental Health and he has a particular interest in working with men individually, in groups and in family situations.

Kerrie James is the Clinical Director of Relationships Australia in New South Wales and has taught and supervised professionals in the area of family and couple therapy since 1980. As a practitioner, Kerrie's interests and publications have been in the area of gender, violence and therapeutic practice. She combines her interests in systemic practice, psychoanalysis and gender in her work with men and boys in family therapy. She is currently involved in research that investigates explanations of men's violence and the implications of these accounts for therapy with perpetrators of domestic violence.

Peter Jones is a lecturer in the School of Social Work and Community Welfare at James Cook University. His interest in gender issues has extended across the areas of education, research and practice, with a particular interest in issues of men and masculinity. He is currently involved in research documenting the perceptions of perpetrators of domestic violence and developing integrated community responses to domestic violence.

Malcolm McCouat is a social worker working in private practice. Until recently he was a lecturer in social work at the University of Queensland. He is very familiar with the experiences of sons whose fathers have been marked by war and other traumas. The way in which psychic and collective defences develop against the vulnerability produced by dangers of various kinds is the starting point in his work with men and with himself.

Fiona McDermott is a senior lecturer in the School of Social Work at the University of Melbourne. She convenes the Mental Health Practice Research Unit in the School and is involved in teaching and supervising research in the mental health field. Her recently published research has focused on work with people with dual psychiatric disabilities and drug and alcohol problems and the development of an evaluation model for use in mental health and drug and alcohol services.

Patrick O'Leary is a lecturer in the School of Social Work and Social Policy at the University of South Australia. Currently, he is completing doctoral research at Flinders University exploring the effects of childhood sexual abuse on men's coping capacities. Patrick has extensive experience as a counsellor in community mental health, family and child welfare and crisis services. In these contexts, he has worked with males who have experienced childhood sexual abuse and men who use violence against women and children.

Elizabeth Ozanne coordinates the Ageing and Long Term Care Research Unit in the School of Social Work at the University of Melbourne. She is involved in teaching in aged policy and program development and has written a number of journal articles, chapters and books. Her latest book, *Ageing and Social Policy in Australia*, was published by Cambridge University Press and jointly edited with Allan Borowski and Sol Encel.

Bob Pease holds a PhD from La Trobe University in Melbourne and is a senior lecturer in Social Work at RMIT University in Melbourne. He has worked in Social Work Education in universities in Tasmania and Victoria since 1980 and has been teaching in the area of men and masculinities since 1989. He is the author of *Men and Sexual Politics: Towards a Profeminist Practice* (Dulwich Centre Publications 1997), co-editor of *Transforming Social Work Practice: Postmodern Critical Perspectives* (Allen & Unwin 1999) and author of *Recreating Men: Postmodern Masculinity Politics* (Sage 2000).

Richard Roberts is a senior lecturer in the School of Social Work at the University of New South Wales in Sydney. In his academic and professional life over the last twenty years, much of his attention has been given to work with gay men and couples. He is author of *Lessons from the Past: Issues for Social Work Theory Today* (Routledge 1990).

1 | Feminism, masculinity politics and the human services

Bob Pease and Peter Camilleri

Feminists in the human services have drawn attention to the prevalence of sexist attitudes and practices in social welfare and, during the last twenty years, female human service workers have developed interventions and policies aimed at overcoming sexism. Feminist practice with women has thus made a significant contribution to critical social work and welfare practice.[1]

It is not surprising that attention has been directed towards women's issues in combating sexism in welfare. The majority of human service workers and the majority of welfare clients are women. However, it is a premise of this book that addressing sexism necessitates an understanding of men as well as women. All human service workers will have contact with men. Furthermore, the majority of the concerns that women bring to welfare workers and counsellors are connected to their relationships with men (Hanmer & Statham 1988).

Although there is a mass of literature in social work and counselling that has much to say about men and masculinities, this is usually done in an implicit and untheorised way. Historically, the study of men has had little place in mainstream human services literature. Feminist social work has not had a lot to say about men either. The key feminist social work texts of the 1980s and 1990s made only passing references to men and there is only one recent feminist text that looks systematically at feminist practice with men.[2]

The contemporary male radical social work literature also neglects analyses of masculinity and practice with men. The focus of the male radical social work literature is on challenging internalised oppression and empowering the disadvantaged; no mention is made of internalised domination.[3] The only exception to this is Keith Pringle's (1995) book in the United Kingdom.

While there has been something of an expansion in the production of texts by men writing about masculinity outside of welfare, most of the studies have either a strongly theoretical orientation[4] or else are focused on men's personal growth.[5] Relatively few of the academic publications by men have focused on practice-oriented issues, while the personal growth books for men tend to ignore issues of gender inequality.

The absence of men in the social work and welfare literature and the neglect of human services practice issues in the masculinities literature is concerning. We are arguing here that the refusal to name men *as men* in social work and the human services limits the potential for challenging gender injustice.

It is timely to develop a critical analysis of men in the human services. This is because a new interest in men and boys is emerging from government at both the policy and service delivery level. For example: men's ill-health has been identified as a major problem and a number of Australian states have now developed draft men's health policies.[6] The causes and consequences of marital separation has led to a new focus on men's ability to maintain relationships.[7] There has also been a growing interest in recent years in developing services for men who are violent to their female partners.[8] The educational attainment of boys is being presented as a major problem, as is violence and bullying in schools.[9] There is also a recognition of a central link between masculinity and crime.[10] Furthermore, at the level of direct practice, male human service workers are becoming increasingly involved in work with men and many feminist workers are also choosing to work with men.

This changing policy and service delivery context presents a number of challenges to social workers and policy-makers. To understand men's relationship to social work and welfare, however, we must analyse men in the context of their broader position in society. Furthermore, changing men in social welfare draws upon similar principles and politics to changing men more generally in society (Hearn 1999, p. 13).

MASCULINITY POLITICS

While feminist social work has been directing attention to the position of women in welfare, a network of men's activities has arisen, including men's support groups, men's ritual healing groups, therapy groups for violent men, programs for boys in schools, men's health programs, fathers' rights groups, courses on men in adult education and academia and profeminist men's social action groups. Some media commentators and writers on masculinity refer to these diverse activities as a 'men's movement'.

There are a variety of ways of classifying this men's movement. For the purpose of our discussion, we identify four distinct approaches: men's rights, mythopoetics, men's liberation and profeminism. These four trends have been the source of considerable conflict in men's politics from its beginning. We briefly outline the main premises of each approach here.[11]

Men's rights

Some men in the men's movement deny that they have power in society and argue that men are more oppressed than women. They express anger at feminism for its challenges to men and they focus their energies on what they see as the relative advantages of women vis-à-vis men. These men comprise the 'men's rights wing' of the men's movement.[12]

A key argument of the men's rights movement is that men are unfairly blamed by women and feminism. Men's rights proponents argue that blaming men for the oppression of women is counterproductive to ending sexism. Goldberg, for example, argues that behaviour arising out of guilt and shame can never be liberating. In his view, blame and guilt are misguided and if the goal is to change men, the strategy is counterproductive (1987, p. 5). The emphasis of much of the men's rights' response to feminism is that women are equally responsible for the problems in the world and the issues confronting them. They are seen to be equally violent, equally sexually aggressive, equally controlling and equally power hungry.

Men's rights advocates sometimes expose the failings of hegemonic masculinity and its effects on men, but they ignore or minimise the effects on women of adhering to this dominant form of masculinity. They also deny the advantages and privileges that men have gained by adopting hegemonic masculinity and they appeal to the tendency within men to regard their own victimisation as most important and to ignore the effect their behaviour has on women (Thorne-Finch 1992, p. 211).

Mythopoetics

The mythopoetic men's movement, first named as such by Shepherd Bliss in 1986, 'looks to ancient mythology and fairy tales, to Jungian and archetypal psychology and to poets and teachers like Robert Bly and James Hillman' (1986, p. 38). Perhaps the most significant single contribution to the development of this movement was Keith Thompson's interview with Robert Bly (1987). Bly elaborated upon his mythical approach in his 1990 bestseller, *Iron John*, and soon after a series of other mythopoetic books followed, including Moore and Gillette (1990), Keen (1991) and Lee (1991).

Bly talks about the importance of men developing 'Zeus energy', which 'encompasses intelligence, robust health, compassionate authority, good will, leadership—in sum, positive power accepted by the male in the service of the community' (Bly 1990, p. 178). Men can get in touch with their male energy by 'learning to visualise the wild man' (1990, p. 179), which involves going back to ancient mythology.

In spite of Bly's claims to the contrary, however, the promotion of the wild man and the warrior has the propensity to reinforce traditional masculinities and entrench oppressive masculine behaviour. Accounts of participants in the mythopoetic men's groups tend to describe patriarchal ways of acting as expressions of their warriorhood (King 1992, p. 137).

In mythopoetic writings, rituals initiating boys into manhood in non-Western cultures are thought to be equally important in the Western context. According to Bly, their absence in Western culture is the major reason why men have such difficulty achieving 'true manhood' (1990, pp. 1–3). Most of these rites of passage for males involve a painful ordeal—beatings, fasting, circumcision or killing an enemy or wild animal and the young men are taught by the elders that men must be able to suffer in silence and be brave (Keen 1991, p. 238). Thus, such initiation rituals not only separate the men from the boys but also the men from the women and many of them are expressions of oppressive social organisation (Samuels 1993, pp. 189–90).

The mythopoetic men's movement is based on an essentialist view of masculinity. Essentialists regard biology as the basic cause of all gender differences. Thus, by construing masculinity as part of that essence, the mythopoetic men's movement concludes that only limited changes in masculinity are desirable and possible. This reinforces traditional masculinity rather than transforming it (King 1992, p. 136). Further, the idea of a masculine essence does not make ethnographic and historical sense as representations of masculinity vary considerably between cultures (Connell 1992, p. 34).

Men's liberation

The mythopoetic men's writings are associated with the wider tradition of men's liberation which is concerned with masculinity therapy and personal growth for men. In this tradition, it is argued that change in men's social relationships with women and with other men will only occur after their inner relationships change. Many writers on masculinity believe that emotional conflicts are the most important issues facing men. Numerous self-help books exist aiming to teach men why and how to feel more deeply. In fact, many men in the men's movement argue that the suppression of feelings is a key factor in the formation of masculinities (Middleton 1992, pp. 119–21).

Pasick defines the problem as men being in a 'deep sleep', which manifests itself in terms of lifestyle imbalances, social isolation, mistrusting of emotions, confusion about dependency/intimacy with women and not taking care of themselves (1992, pp. 10–17). Steiner refers to 'emotional illiteracy' to describe men not knowing their own emotions or what causes them (1986, p. 112), whilst Biddulph identifies men's major difficulty as isolation, reflected in loneliness, compulsive competition and life-long timidity (1994, p. 4).

Other men's liberation writers refer to the notion of men's woundedness. Farmer, for instance, talks about men as the 'walking wounded'. These wounds can be inflicted at any time in a man's life, but Farmer regards childhood injuries as the ones that have the most significant impact. They are the wounds resulting from sexual abuse, from physical or verbal battering, or from the absence of intimacy with father or mother (1991, p. 4). Most of the associated therapeutic approaches involve the search for childhood precedents of our current tragedies (Kupers 1993, p. 142).

Kreiner argues that men 'behave oppressively towards women because they are scared' (1992, p. 52) and Orkin similarly asserts that men's violence is a result of the abuses they suffer (1991, p. 9). Men do suffer, but this suffering cannot justify men's treatment of other people (Middleton 1992, p. 125). Small boys may not be fully responsible for the choices they make but grown men continue to exercise their choices largely for the benefits they receive (Jukes 1993, p. 136), however unconscious the link.

We do not believe that personal or spiritual change will address the problems of exploitation and power inequality. By focusing solely on personal change, there is seen to be no need to change economic and social structures and men settle for an individualistic solution (Kaufman 1993, pp. 271–2). This seems inevitable when most personal growth and spiritual paths promise individual liberation and fulfilment, irrespective of social and economic conditions.

We do not wish to argue that there is no place for personal change and healing in the transformation of men. Unfortunately, few men seem to have used insights gained from therapy or personal healing as a basis for political action. Nevertheless, it is important that we continue to explore the relationship between men's psyche and the material and social world, for this will enable us more adequately to address the relationship between personal change in men's subjectivities and simultaneous change in the social relations of gender dominance.

Profeminism

Profeminist men stress the importance of men working as allies with women in a struggle to transform hegemonic masculinity and patriarchal relations of dominance. Profeminism for men involves a sense of responsibility to our own and other men's sexism, and a commitment to work with women to end men's violence (Douglas 1993). It acknowledges that men benefit from the oppression of women, drawing men's attention to the privileges we receive as men and the harmful effects these privileges have on women (Thorne-Finch 1992, p. 234).

A profeminist perspective explains dominant masculinity in structural and cultural terms. From this perspective, for men to change, we have to reconstruct masculinity in ways that acknowledge its social dimension. That means challenging gender inequality in the public arena. As men, it is important that we confront our political position. We cannot just relinquish the reality of social power. We have to develop a conscious politics aimed at creating new laws, new values and new organisational forms. It is not enough to bring a new man into existence. We have to reconstruct the whole gender order (Cockburn 1988, p. 32). This means challenging the masculinism of trade unions, political parties and social movements. It means openly supporting anti-discrimination policies and campaigns against sexual harassment and sexual assault, as well as acting against patriarchy through the creation of anti-sexist groups and networks (Hearn 1987, pp. 168–70).

Men Against Sexual Assault (MASA) is an example of pro-feminist politics in Australia. MASA has been involved in the organisation of forums on issues like pornography, militarism, sexual harassment and rape, conducting workshops in schools on anti-sexist masculinity for boys, producing newsletters, running workshops and giving public talks educating men about the impact of patriarchy on women's lives, speaking out in the public media about the objectification of women and organising marches and the White Ribbon Campaign against men's violence.[13]

Profeminists recognise that sexism has an impact on men as well as women. To oppress others, it is necessary to suppress oneself. Systemic male dominance deforms men too, as evidenced in stress-related illnesses and emotional inexpressiveness. Further-more, of course, not all men benefit equally from the operation of the structures of domination. Issues of race, sexuality, class, disability and age significantly affect the extent to which men benefit from patriarchy.

RATIONALE AND PURPOSES OF THE BOOK

While the contributors to this book all draw upon a diverse range of theoretical frameworks in their work with men, all of them are influenced by feminist and profeminist principles in their practice. No attempt is made in this book to present a unified feminist or profeminist perspective.

One of the aims of this book is to redress the invisibility of men within the social work and human services literature and to describe some of the work at present being undertaken with men. A major objective is to introduce those interested in developing new approaches to working with men to a variety of models and contexts in which such practice takes place. The contributors outline the rationale for, and the content of, their work with men. They describe the work that has been undertaken, how it is delivered, the difficulties and dangers associated with it, together with an indication of what it can achieve. We hope that by compiling these contributions, the book will stimulate further innovative work in these areas.

This book is equally concerned with men and masculinity in relation to both those who provide welfare services as well as those who receive them. Social work and other human service jobs are classified as female occupations unless one becomes a manager, an administrator or a researcher. Caring is regarded by most men as a non-masculine activity. However, some men do enter social work and helping professions to work directly with people. Why do these men choose to enter social work and counselling? Do they see this work differently to women? We know very little about male social workers and counsellors and about the extent to which they give any priority to developing an anti-sexist culture in their work with men.

OVERVIEW

The book is divided into four parts. Part I explores some of the gender issues facing workers in the human services. Part II examines a range of gender-based practice frameworks in working with men as service users. Part III outlines different practice approaches for working with male offenders. Part IV addresses ways of responding to social difference and inequality in men's lives.

The first section begins with Bob Pease's chapter in which he identifies some of the theoretical issues and political dilemmas in working with men in the human services. Drawing upon critical theoretical explorations of masculinities, he emphasises the importance of locating men's lives within the context of patriarchy, hegemonic masculinity, and the social divisions between men.

While women have numerically dominated the human services, men have tended to be disproportionately represented in senior positions. In Chapter 3 Peter Camilleri and Peter Jones examine the contradictions faced by those men who undertake caring roles within a patriarchal discourse which has structured women's and men's work in the human services.

Part II begins with a chapter by Kerrie James who presents an understanding of men and masculinity by emphasising the role of men's relationships and attachments to significant others. She demonstrates how adherence to traditional aspects of masculinity promotes men's and boys' disconnection from themselves and alienation from others. Using case examples, she outlines the implications of an attachment framework for working with men in families.

In the next chapter, Mark Furlong explores the issues involved in engaging men in counselling. He emphasises the importance of avoiding both collision and collusion in work with men and demonstrates how relevant language and the use of positioning can elicit a constructive rather than an adversarial dynamic.

In Chapter 6 Mal McCouat argues that one of the causes and effects of the exploitative behaviour of men is the defensive acting out of vulnerability. He demonstrates the process of supporting and challenging male clients to reclaim their consciousness of vulnerability, to take responsibility for it and to identify and nurture it in others.

Chapter 7 by Patrick O'Leary explores theoretical considerations and practical ways of working with men who have experienced childhood sexual abuse. He identifies some of the difficulties that these men may face in the current social and political context and describes how, for men who have been subject to sexual abuse, dominant constructions of masculinity can contribute to the silencing of their experience and to stories of self-blame. He also outlines a number of therapeutic themes in working with men on these issues.

In the final chapter in this section, Peter Humphries reflects on his experience of counselling men with a psychiatric disability, with a particular focus on engaging these men in a therapeutic relationship. He outlines the implications of an anti-oppressive approach to counselling and identifies approaches he has found helpful in developing trust with men.

The four chapters in Part III explore the challenges of working with men's violence and criminality. In the first chapter in this section, Mary Hood examines how a side effect of the feminist construction of child abuse and child protection has been to cast a shadow over the interactions of all men with all children, creating real dilemmas for men in child protection work and for men in families. She argues that rather than just preventing men from contact with children, child protection policy and practice needs to work to find safe and explicit ways to better include men in family, therapeutic and community relationships with children.

In Chapter 10 Rob Hall describes pitfalls and challenges in working with men who have been violent to their intimate partners. He describes ways of encouraging men to challenge masculine ways of thinking and practices that contribute to abuse and emphasises the importance of safety, responsibility, respect and accountability in work with men.

In the Australian juvenile justice system, 90 per cent of the young people under community supervision or custodial care are males aged between fifteen and eighteen years. In Chapter 11 Mark Griffiths demonstrates how male workers in criminal justice are responding to the challenges of gender-based crime and how they are searching for more effective paradigms of practice. He explores possible future directions arising from the development of restorative justice conferences.

The link between masculinity and adult crime is also well established, with men comprising 95 per cent of the Australian prison population. In Chapter 12 David Rose discusses the wider social factors that impact on men who commit crimes, including unemployment, educational attainment, capacity to maintain effective relationships, substance abuse, disabilities and general confusion about men's role and place in a changing society. He also examines some of the issues and dilemmas inherent in social work practice with men in a prison context.

The four chapters in Part IV examine issues of social difference and inequality in men's lives. The focus of Chapter 13 by Fiona McDermott and Elizabeth Ozanne is on those issues relating to the utilisation of and access to health and welfare services of men in the 60-plus age group. They discuss the adequacy of service system responses to older men and address the implications of these issues for social work practice with older men.

In Chapter 14 Graham Atkinson, in an interview with Bob Pease, demonstrates how historical processes have devalued the Indigenous male role in both the family and the community. Many Indigenous men have embraced alcoholism and become the recipients of welfare, while family violence, unemployment, ill-health and substance abuse continue to be significant problems in the Indigenous community. Graham describes how a newly formed Indigenous Men's Business Movement is beginning to tackle these issues by discussing ways of challenging men's violence and promoting men's health and wellbeing in Indigenous communities.

Chapter 15 by Richard Roberts examines the fluidity of gender identity and sexual orientation and the implications for social work practice with gay identified men. Practitioner self-awareness is an important issue and he warns practitioners of the dangers of confusing gender and sexual orientation. Richard concludes the chapter by identifying common problems faced by gay men, including 'coming out', achieving intimacy, and dealing with homophobia.

In the final chapter Steve Golding challenges heterosexual practitioners to confront their own homophobia. He argues that the invisibility of heterosexual dominance has meant that many human service agencies do not address the issue of homophobia in their work with men. By challenging heterosexual dominance and homophobia, he argues, we not only address the oppression of specific groups of men, but also contribute to a society that accepts and celebrates the differences in all of us.

Practice with men in the human services can either reinforce or oppose masculinisation. We believe that men, as well as women, in the human services have a part to play in reducing or eliminating sexism. We see the beginnings of a new agenda for feminist and profeminist practice with men developing and we hope that this book will make an important contribution to that agenda.

PART I

GENDER ISSUES FACING
WORKERS IN THE
HUMAN SERVICES

2 | Theoretical issues and political dilemmas in working with men

Bob Pease

The aim of this chapter is to highlight some of the theoretical issues and political dilemmas involved in working with men in the human services. To develop a framework for practice with men, we have to adequately conceptualise the issues facing men. These are confusing and unsettling times for many men. To make sense of this confusion it is important to understand men's experiences within the context of the patriarchal structures in society and their relationship to class, race and gender regimes. Men and women who work with men in the human services should have an analysis of the social construction of masculinities and they need to understand how the forces that construct dominant masculinities embed men and women in relations of dominance and subordination that limit the potential for them to be in partnership with each other.

To the extent that we ignore the social construction of masculinity, it blocks insight into the real trouble in men's lives. Furthermore, if men do not grasp the basic notion of gender as a social construction, then feminist critiques of patriarchy, dominant masculinity and abusive male behaviours are going to be felt by men at a deeply personal level (Schwalbe 1996, pp. 187, 231).

UNSETTLING MEN

Although, of course, there are differences in emphasis, there seems to be general agreement that the central features of traditional masculinity are: emotional stoicism, homophobia, emphasis on work and achievement, competitiveness, distant fathering, neglect of health needs and mistrust of women (Brooks 1991, p. 52). It is also becoming apparent that women are less accepting of these features of traditional masculinity.

One-third of all marriages in Australia end in divorce. Research demonstrates that resentments and disputes over the various forms of marital inequality and abuse of women are among the factors men and women cite as contributing to the breakdown of their marriages (Dempsey 1997, p. 226). Thus, it would seem that most marital breakdown is directly related to men's sense of marital entitlement and their sexism. It is clear that in spite of their relatively advantageous position, many men feel disadvantaged compared to women. Farrell (1993) argues that if men do not feel powerful, then they are not powerful. He reduces power to a psychological issue and many men identify with this position. If they don't *feel* like powerful patriarchs then the feminist analysis must be wrong. This then leads to a blindness to the institutional power of men (Schwalbe 1996, p. 149) and a lack of awareness of how many of the disadvantages suffered by men are part of a political system that substantially benefits the majority of men (Sterba 1998, p. 297).

Men often want things to change but they do not want to relinquish their power. A feminist-informed approach to working with men challenges the distribution of power in families and encourages men to rethink their power. This means, as Connell has suggested, disrupting men's settled ways of thinking (1987, p. xii).

Many of the beliefs men hold are the cause of the troubles in their lives. Thus, the starting point for work with men is to assess their beliefs. What beliefs does the man hold about masculinity? What are the sources of these beliefs? How are these beliefs associated with the difficulties the man is experiencing? What are the potential harmful effects of these beliefs (Allen & Gordon 1990, p. 138)?

Men's socialisation leads to the individual beliefs that can promote abusive behaviours (Russell 1995). Mederos argues that all men are embedded in a personal patriarchal system and that all men share to some extent a sense of entitlement to make normative claims on women. The differences among men relate to the claims they make and how they attempt to enforce them (1987, p. 43). Thus, although men's use of power and control is central in work with violent men, I believe that it is an issue in work with all men.

Men need to be helped to acknowledge their tendencies to act oppressively and they should be assisted to devise strategies to change dominating behaviour. They should also be encouraged to develop wider repertoires of behaviour and models of masculinity not associated with violence, control and objectification (Pringle 1995, pp. 153–4).

THE LIMITS OF SEX ROLE THEORY IN UNDERSTANDING MEN

The main theoretical framework that informs work with men in the human services is sex role theory. The sex role approach to masculinity utilises the theoretical ideas underlying liberal femi-nism, wherein women's disadvantages are said to result from stereotypical customary expectations, internalised by both men and women.

Sex role theory informed the early men's liberation movement of the 1970s, whose theorists maintained that freeing sex role conventions might also be good for men as well as women. Thus, men were encouraged to 'break . . . out of the straight-jacket of sex roles' (Farrell 1975, p. 8) and 'to free themselves of the sex-role stereotypes that limit their ability to be human' (Sawyer 1974, p. 170). The implication was that men could transform themselves without reference to wider social processes, the male role being something we could dispose of, allowing the human being in the man to emerge.

One of the major limitations of sex role theory is that it under-emphasises the economic and political power that men exercise over women. Male and female roles are seen to be equal, thus enabling men and women to engage in a common cause against sex role oppression.

What is consistently missing in sex role theory is a recognition of the extent to which men's gender identities are based upon a struggle for social power. Men clearly suffer from adhering to dominant forms of masculinity. Many men are now concluding that the social and political gains of having power over women do not outweigh the physical, social and psychological health costs incurred (Newman 1997, p. 137). Most men, however, approve and support the overall system in spite of the burdens and they simply want more benefits and less burdens (Ball 1997, p. 71). There is no evidence that liberating men from the traditional male sex role will lead to men relinquishing their privilege and social power. And yet this is where traditional approaches to understanding and working with men are often heading.[1] Traditional approaches to working with men attempt to address the needs of male clients. However, to the extent that work with men enables men to be more effective, it may also enable them to be more dominant (Rowan 1997, p. 14). The focus on men's concerns and their needs for self-acceptance and resolution of their problems contributes to men not taking women's concerns seriously. Men's reality is given paramount status (Schwalbe 1996, p. 193). I believe that work with men has to be informed by feminism and the lived experience of women.

THE PORTRAYAL OF MEN AS A HOMOGENEOUS GROUP

In some feminist social work texts, however, all men are seen as a coherent 'gender class' with the same vested interests in controlling women. Some radical feminists believe that men will never change and that their dominance is inevitable (Segal 1987, p. 17). Within this perspective, there is no basis for men to change. If all men are the enemy, then it is difficult to envisage the possibility of men and women working together against patriarchy (Edley & Wetherell 1995, p. 196). If all men are innately violent and controlling, there is little optimism for change.

How meaningful is it to talk about men as a homogeneous group? When it is said that men control the mode of reproduction and that men dominate women in the public sphere, does this mean *all* men? Are all men violent? Are all men potential rapists?

One of the problems with this categorical approach to men is that it makes oppression definitional of men. It implies that men oppress women by virtue of being men. Men do not all benefit equally from the operation of the structures of domination. Issues of race, sexuality, class, disability and age affect the extent to which men benefit from the patriarchal dividend. While the gender hierarchy involves men's domination of women, it also includes a system of internal dominance in which a minority of men dominate the majority of men (Sabo & Gordon 1995, p. 10).

A categorical approach to men can also be used to obscure *some* men's privilege. In the presentation of men's health statistics, for example, there is often little consideration of social divisions between men. So although the health status and life chances of some men in the gender order are advantaged, other sub-groups of men are systematically disadvantaged. Aboriginal men's health, the health of men from low socioeconomic groups, gay men and disabled men etc. are disregarded in most discussions of men's health (Wadham 1997, p. 21).

We are now entering a new stage in which variations among men are seen as central to the understanding of men's lives (Kimmel & Messner 1989, p. 9). So, we cannot speak of masculinity as a singular term but rather should explore masculinities. Men are as socially diverse as women and this diversity entails differences between men in relation to class, ethnicity, age, sexuality, bodily facility, religion, world views, parental/marital status, occupation and propensity for violence (Collinson 1992, p. 35).

Differences are also found across cultures and through historical time. The discourse about 'masculinity' is constructed out of 5 per cent of the world's population of men, in one region of the world, at one moment in history. We know from ethnographic work in different cultures how non-Western masculinities can be very different from the Western norm (Connell 1991, p. 3).[2]

MEN DOING FEMINISM

Is it possible for men to engage in practices that serve women's interests? It is generally agreed that men cannot be feminists because we do not have women's experience (Reinharz 1992, pp. 14–15). However, can men engage in profeminist practice if they can fulfil certain conditions? Or are we locked into an ontological position within patriarchy because of our location in the social structure?

I believe that men *can* change in the direction of feminism. Men have choices as to whether they accept patriarchy or work collectively against it. Before men can organise collectively, though, they must transform their subjectivities and practices. I believe that there are spaces in patriarchy for men 'to appreciate the possibilities of being different and being against sexism and against patriarchy' (Hearn 1992, p. 19).

Although we cannot individually or as a group escape our material position in patriarchy, I believe that we can change our ideological and discursive position. I draw upon feminist standpoint theory here.[3] The advantage of the notion of standpoint is that it relates to both structural location as well as the discursive construction of subjectivity, allowing us to distinguish between a traditional 'men's standpoint' and a 'profeminist men's standpoint'.

A traditional men's standpoint is based on the privileges and powers men have, and excludes the perspective of women. A profeminist men's standpoint involves an ability to be critical of men's position in society and how it contributes to the inequality of women as well as developing an ethical and moral commitment to addressing that inequality and discrimination because of the harm it causes (May 1998, pp. 342–6).[4]

Thus I believe that it is possible for men to change their subjectivities and practices to constitute a profeminist men's standpoint. The process of change is itself a requirement in formulating a profeminist men's standpoint. Men have to change their vantage point if they want to see the world from a different position and this entails more than just a theoretical shift. It also requires men to actively engage in profeminist struggles in both the private and public arenas.

Men have access to some areas of male behaviour and thought that women do not have. In this sense, women cannot know the 'content of the deliberate strategies that men and male dominated institutions use to maintain their power' (Kelly et al. 1994, p. 33). Profeminist men can use their position to gain insights into how men construct themselves in a dominant position. And, given that men value masculine authority more highly, they should use it to resocialise men.

On the other hand, there are dangers when men engage with feminist issues. Feminist scholarship is sometimes taken more seriously when men discuss it than when women do. There is also a danger that men will claim a place in feminism and that the dominance of men will assert itself on feminist knowledge as a right.

Women will also bring to this issue their own individual experiences of men which will range from loving intimacy to violence and abuse. It is likely that women will continue to be divided between those who will work with men and those who will not. However, while many women continue to be sceptical about men's involvement with feminism, a shift in opinion is occurring that is opening up possibilities for profeminist men and women to work together within a broader feminist movement.

ENGAGING MEN IN CHANGE: SELF-INTEREST OR ETHICS?

How do we best engage men in the process of change? There is a major division in masculinity politics between those who argue that men should change for enlightened self-interest reasons and those who advocate change on the basis of an ethical or moral position. For those who argue the enlightened self-interest position, it is said that to oppress others, it is necessary to suppress oneself and that systemic male dominance not only oppresses women, it deforms men as well; for example, men, more than women, die of stress-related illness and violence and have a shorter life expectancy (Cockburn 1991, p. 222).

Some even go so far as to suggest that men's everyday masculine identities are afflicted with psychopathology. It is suggested that men's laconicism, hot and cold emotional responses, stoical defences against unmet needs, compulsive action-driven grandiosity or omnipotence and refusal to acknowledge sickness, injury and incapacity, constitute a form of borderline personality disorder (Ball 1997, pp. 27, 70).

It is true that patriarchy distorts men's lives as well as women's lives. Many men feel grief and have been victimised as boys. One has to ask, though, in what ways would a men's movement, organised around men's enlightened self-interests, advance women's struggles? The risk in arguing that it is in men's interests to change is that men may adopt a strategy that benefits them, rather than focusing on overcoming the oppression of women. Furthermore, the issue of personal exploration as opposed to activism is a contentious one. Does changing oneself as a man help to challenge patriarchy at the structural level? Does personal change in particular men's practices undermine patriarchal relations?

For those who advocate the ethical and moral position, it is said that if men want to liberate themselves from 'the male malaise', they will have to let go of male privilege, rather than engaging in intrapsychic self-affirmation. Men have to 'come to understand the injustice that has been done to women' (Ruether 1992, pp. 14–15) and they must acknowledge the injustice of their historical privilege as men.

bell hooks (1992, pp. 13–14) is critical of the view that it is only when those in power understand how they too have been victimised, that they will rebel against the structures of domination. She says that 'individuals of great privilege who are in no way victimised are capable via political choices of working on behalf of the oppressed'. Thus, one can reject domination through ethical and political understanding. And, of course, it is important to acknowledge that, throughout history, men have taken principled stands on women's rights.[5]

However, how does one articulate a moral stance that challenges men to consider the social justice implications of their behaviour in the world without alienating them? Understanding the experiences of an oppressed group does not appear to be sufficient, unless it involves 'some kind of transformation experience, particularly of the sort that results in the unsettling of the person's self and position' (Babbitt 1993, p. 256).

I do not see these strategies as being antithetical to each other. I think that men's interests can be reconstructed in ways that include a moral ethic. I believe that men have a stake in an egalitarian future and that feminism can enhance men's lives. So I see it as being very important to communicate how feminism is in men's interests; interests in transcending gender hierarchy rather than interests in taking a bigger piece of the pie (Brod 1998, p. 200).

It is feminist analyses that offer models of relationships based on mutuality rather than dominance (Ganley 1990, p. 25). Pence and Paymar, in contrast to their power and control wheel, which describes men's violence, have developed an equality wheel that includes economic partnership, shared responsibility, responsible parenting, honesty and accountability, trust and support, respect, non-threatening behaviour and negotiation and fairness (1993, p. 94).

Research shows that egalitarian couples have better communication than other couples and that both men and women are more satisfied in their relationships (Rabin 1996, p. 46). Such couples define equality in their relationships in three ways: a subjective appraisal of the level of fairness in the relationship, an equal balance of power in decision-making and equal sharing of household and parenting roles (Rabin 1996, p. 56). If we can help men see that new forms of partnership with women offer men more positive

and fulfilling relationships, they may be more willing to let go of
dominating and controlling behaviours.

MOVING BEYOND THE AGENCY–STRUCTURE DUALISM

To address these issues, however, we need to understand more fully
how hegemonic masculinity 'gets into' men and how men might
come to work for these changes. What are the mechanisms through
which men's personality and masculinity come to reflect the gender
relations of patriarchy? We need to understand the ways in which
dominant ideology is internalised in the psyches of men and how
this ideology interacts with material conditions to shape men's
experience.

Without a conceptual framework encompassing and reflecting
the relationship between the lived experience of men and the
institutional structures in which they are embedded, the possibilities
for transforming men's lives and the social relations of gender are
doubtful. One either ends up in despair, immobilised by an overly
socially determined self or one posits a voluntarist and idealist view
of how men can change, ignoring the material and social basis of
patriarchy.

It is here that I think that the postmodern interrogation of
critical theory is of most importance. From a postmodern critical
perspective, masculinity is not an inherent property of individuals.
Rather, we learn the discursive frameworks and work out how to
position ourselves 'correctly' as male (Davies 1989, p. 13). Within
these frameworks we are invited to take up or turn down different
subject positions and a sense of masculine identity that goes with
them. That is, each framework enables men to think of themselves
as men in particular ways (Jackson 1990, p. 286). Such a perspective
enables us to identify that the supposedly fixed position between
anatomical sexuality and gender stereotypes can be broken. We are
thus more able to legitimate behaviours that do not seem to derive
from one's biological sex.

Through the recognition of a possible multiplicity of identities
for men, we are able to challenge the view that it is not in men's
interests to change. Men's interests can be reconstructed by men
repositioning themselves in the patriarchal discourse and by men
constructing alternative profeminist subject positions.[6]

AVOIDING COLLUSION WITH MEN

When men work with men it is important that they recognise their kinship with fellow men. However, the common elements that exist between male workers and male clients present a number of problems. There is a fine line between emphasising the commonalities between men and men colluding with oppressive attitudes and behaviours (Pringle 1995, p. 215). When Bathrick and Kaufman audio-taped group sessions with violent men for their female supervisors, the women identified ways in which the male workers did not confront assumptions of privilege and dominance (1990, p. 113). If we do not challenge men's abusive and sexist behaviour, we are colluding with that behaviour. This is a problem for relations between men more generally.

In light of these dangers, how confronting should we be with other men? How do we invite men to examine their behaviour without increasing their resistance? If we confront oppressive attitudes and behaviour too strongly, we may lose the engagement of the man being confronted. However, if we do not confront sufficiently, then we may well be colluding. Men should never act in a way that condones men's victimisation of women and supports their demands for patriarchal entitlement (Brooks 1998, p. 79). At the same time, we have to connect with men's experience. The only way through this dilemma is for men to critically reflect upon their own socialisation processes and engage with their own gendered subjectivity.[7]

Work with men in the human services should be one aspect of a broader strategy for changing unequal power relations between women and men. To address this issue, we need to encourage the construction of new frameworks for profeminist practice with men in social work and welfare. In my view such frameworks have to acknowledge and grapple with the theoretical issues and political dilemmas that I have identified in this chapter.

3 | Doing 'women's work'?: Men, masculinity and caring

Peter Camilleri and Peter Jones

In this chapter we explore some of the issues concerning men working in the human services. It is an area that has traditionally been seen as women's work and there has been a significant gendered pattern of employment (see Christie 1998). Men are clustered in certain areas of practice and in particular positions such as management. This is not a new phenomenon and has been a major issue of debate in the last 35 years (see Lawrence 1965; Walton 1975; Camilleri 1996; Christie 1998). In addressing these issues, we examine the labour force participation in the community service sector; the issues of gender in the construction of 'care' (in particular how patriarchal discourse has structured the possibilities of men's and women's work); and issues and contradictions of men who remain in direct practice.

The human services include areas such as nursing, teaching, social work, psychology and the myriad of allied health professions and social welfare paraprofessionals. This chapter is mainly concerned with those areas that come under the heading of social welfare; that is, social work, welfare work, community work and so on. Traditionally, the human services sector has been seen as somewhat peripheral to the 'real' economy. However, the tremendous growth of community services and recognition of the important role which this sector plays in the economy has meant that governments, policy-makers and researchers have increasingly realised that the sector is no longer peripheral, but rather central to many people's lives as both workers and consumers of services.

The Australian Bureau of Statistics' 1996 survey found the sector involves over 8000 businesses and organisations with 321 000 employees and an expenditure of $9.7 billion (ABS 1996). Welfare expenditure now consumes the major proportion of the Australian Federal Government's budget each year (approximately $50 billion).

The sector has also been identified in recent times as an area of expanding occupational growth and employment demand (for example, see Department of Employment Education and Training 1991). Certainly in the 1990s DEET had predicted that the fastest growing occupations and professions would be psychology, social work and to a smaller extent welfare work. It was expected that from 1991–2001, psychology would grow by 93 per cent, social work 83.1 per cent and welfare work by 53.8 per cent. The other major professions such as teaching and nursing were expected to grow by only 25.6 per cent and 20.5 per cent respectively (DEET 1991).

These predictions of an expanding sector with increasing employment opportunities are often at odds with practitioners' perceptions of cutbacks and dwindling resources. However, for the purposes of this chapter, our interest is in the gendered nature of the workforce in the human services sector, and men's position within that workforce, now and into the future.

It is a truism that the human services are dominated numerically by women and that most of the clients of the human services are also women. This feminisation of both the providers and consumers of services has been noted by many commentators (see Christie 1998; Martin 1990 and 1996; Martin & Healy 1993). Yet despite the numerical dominance of women in the sector, there is clear evidence of a reproduction of the patriarchal relations of wider society when the position of men in the sector is considered.

For example, men in the human services tend to have significantly different career paths to their female counterparts. It has been noted many times by feminists that while there may be fewer men than women in nursing, primary school teaching, social work, etc., they tend to dominate senior management positions and they reach management levels much more quickly than women. Career paths for men also tend to be characterised by continuous employment, mainly fulltime, in relatively secure positions.

In addition to differences in career prospects, American research on social work in particular has indicated that there are also

considerable pay differentials between men and women (Huber &
Orlando 1995; Gibelman & Schervish 1995). Over the decades,
there have been calls for more men in many of these professions
as a mechanism for increasing status and pay (see Lawrence 1965).
The European Commission and the Equal Opportunities Commission (United Kingdom) have also called for the employment of
more men in social work and other similar occupations (Christie
1998).

CARE AND GENDER

Pringle (1995) points out that this gendered nature of social welfare
organisations can be witnessed with respect to both vertical and
horizontal segregation. Vertical segregation refers to the fact that
men tend to gravitate quickly towards managerial positions within
organisations while more women remain in direct care positions.
Horizontal segregation occurs when men move to particular fields
within the sector, often areas of practice that are seen as having
higher status or are more explicitly concerned with issues of
control. Explanations for this gender segregation have tended to
focus on a number of factors, including the reproduction within
the sector of wider patriarchal norms, the nature of the discourse
of caring and its relationship to the notion of 'women's work',
and the relationship of various masculinities to an occupation that
is characterised by stereotypically feminine concerns.

The notion of the 'caring' professions (Hugman 1991), and of
caring itself, produces a powerful discourse, which creates images
of love, affection, self-sacrifice and intimacy. This notion of care
is embedded within the discourse of femininity. In this sense,
professions such as nursing and social work are not just seen as
women's professions but the actual tasks undertaken by them are
seen as women's tasks. Women are defined as carers not in any
abstract sense but in their everyday work as mothers, sisters,
daughters and workers. Women provide care bounded with notions
of love, obligation and duty. Care is a 'labour of love' (Graham
1983, p. 15).

Nursing and social work in particular are seen to be constituted
in the skills viewed as in some ways 'natural' feminine characteristics. These professions have battled to have their worth and
specialised knowledge and skills recognised. However, in everyday
discourse there is a sense in which most women 'nurse' and 'social

work' others. Caring for others becomes part of women's self-identity and their sense of self. Relationships with others are predicated on the sense of care, so that women 'care' for children, husbands and fathers, as an integral part of their social relationships. It is this, argues Graham (1983), that provides the special space for women in a patriarchal world and discourse. In a patriarchal society it therefore follows that caring will often be undervalued and ignored (Bryson 1992).

Feminists such as Ungerson (1983), Graham (1983), and Finch and Groves (1983) argue that 'care' has a number of distinct meanings and, in particular, they distinguished between caring about and caring for someone. These distinctions are useful in shedding light on the relationship of men to the discourse of caring.

'Caring about' is an intellectual activity. It does not denote intimacy but rather the opposite—abstractness and objectivity. There is no personal involvement and it denotes a sense of professionalism. Such a concept would see that danger for many professionals lies in being too close and personal with their clients. Caring about has a sense of objectivity and not friendship. The human service sector has traditionally being stratified into areas that provide for close and intimate contact with clients and those more removed from this degree of intimacy. Much of the work is stratified with the higher status professions having little personal contact and intimacy with service users. It can be argued that there is a hierarchy within the human service sector and professions and that within this hierarchy those professions which provide a space for the client to be seen within a context of formality and objectivity are deemed more professional.

Caring about, therefore, seems to be embedded with a language that is similar to the descriptions of masculinity. It is a language in which power and control are central themes. This provides an argument for caring about to be seen as a masculine activity. This construction allows for the discourse of management and policy analysis to exclude women and to ascribe higher value and status to the parts of the human services sector in which men are more likely to be found.

On the other hand, 'caring for' involves intimate and personal relationships with another. Those professions that are characterised by caring for involve the actual tasks of care.

What is different is that caring work involves a degree of intimacy, of closeness socially (emotionally and/or physically) between the carer and the cared-for. Moreover, it requires the professional to recognise, even to make central in theory and practice, the individuality of the person receiving the service (Hugman 1991, p. 15).

Such care, as 'women's task' is subsequently devalued and ascribed significantly lower status within the sector, and this status often translates directly into lower pay, less secure positions and fewer opportunities for career advancement.

It has been argued here that the discourse of 'care' provides for a reading of 'caring for' as essentially a defining dimension of women's identity, a reading that serves to lock them into patriarchal structures and into a prescribed identity as 'natural' carers. It is a discourse that appears to exclude men. Men on the other hand are identified with 'caring about' where judgments are made on the basis of male 'rationality' and 'logic'. This accounts for the segmentation within the human services where men are more likely to end up in positions associated with the allocation of resources and issues of power and control.

CHALLENGES AND OPPORTUNITIES

The feminist analysis is extremely powerful in its explanation of this gendered separation of caring work into the managing and allocating of resources on the one hand and the provision of the actual care services on the other. What is more difficult is explaining the existence of men who choose to work in direct practice areas that are characterised by a 'caring for' rather than a 'caring about' ethos.

Many men deliberately choose to work in direct care roles. There may be many reasons for such a choice, but there is no doubt that this situation has the potential to represent a challenge to traditional models of masculinity and to create both issues and opportunities for the men involved. This section will examine a range of issues for men in human service work and explore the ways in which the conscious use of gender in practice creates an opportunity for male workers to contribute to the challenging of masculine stereotypes and the reduction of sexism.

As previously noted, men in human service work as in most forms of paid work, have privileged spaces. Their work is constructed as a career and their identity is bound up with being a worker. Identity for women workers is typically meshed with being partners, mothers, daughters and so on. For men, work has been their identity. This privileged space is being challenged by feminists and offers male workers an opportunity to move beyond the stereotype. It demands that male workers construct their identity not through work but through being connected to a web of relationships (see Gilligan 1982). This challenges men to see themselves within the context of their privileged position within society.

Social work as one of the professions within human services has consciously challenged the hegemony of masculinity. For many male practitioners the feminist movement has opened the debate on what constitutes masculinity. It has allowed for male social workers in particular to argue that masculinity needs to be constructed within a continuum and not as a dichotomised category. This allows for *masculinities* and it provides space for male practitioners to construct a different discourse on practice. This discourse does not see 'caring' as a natural feminine characteristic but as part of a patriarchal discourse that has locked women into particular types of work.

Stereotypically, care by male workers has often been seen in the context of sexuality. Males who care are, it seems, different. Sensitivity and the actual tasks of caring for are segregated out of hegemonic masculinity. For masculinity in this culture 'real' men do not do 'women's work'. Those who do provide 'care' have to be accounted for. The accounts range from redefining the work to questioning the sexuality of the worker.

It has been noted (Pringle 1998) that social work is a self-reflective social practice and male social workers engage and are engaged in the contradictions of a gendered activity. Feminist criticisms are 'part and parcel' of social work education. The focus on anti-sexist and anti-discriminatory practice has the potential of sensitising male social workers. This needs, however, to be translated into practice. For male social workers this involves being aware of the discriminating structures of society and being engaged in practices that do not reinforce those structures. It is also to be personally cognisant of privileged and taken-for-granted assumptions of power.

The growth of the men's movement during the 1980s and 1990s has raised particular issues for practitioners. For many men, engagement in men's issues is not central to their practice. The radical literature in social welfare has focused on challenging oppression. Numerous texts on anti-oppressive practice draw on a discourse that is focused on the disadvantaged and the structural

changes needed (see Ife 1997; Mullaly 1997). The internal contradictions of oppression and domination have not been explored.

The lenses of gender, ethnicity, race and class are used to
explore the problematic world. They are, however, not used to
focus on human service practice itself. Gender and social welfare
has essentially been a debate around the issues facing women both
as clients and as practitioners. Feminist social work literature, for
example, has not explored issues facing men both as clients and as
practitioners (with one exception, see Cavanagh & Cree 1996). In
much of the literature, the practice itself has not been critically
examined in relationship to gender. Many of the texts, while
focusing on gender issues, seem to make the practitioner 'gender
neutral'. The way women and men practitioners work needs to be
deconstructed. The question needs to be raised, is practice itself
gendered? Do women and men practitioners work differently and
if so, how and in what ways?

The development of a range of services, support groups and
programs for boys and men (see Pease 1997) is an outcome of
contradictory forces. They are a product of both genuine concern
and, in some cases, they are also a backlash against the threat of
feminism. With the latter we are seeing the emergence of arguments concerning power and privilege that are associated with men.
The notion of patriarchal dominance is being seriously questioned
by many men's groups who see women as having taken up power
and position and believe that men's rights have been diminished.
Certain men's groups argue that men's rights are being eroded.
Development of men's services in areas of health and the proposed
establishment of a men's shelter for abused husbands in an Australian city appear to be arguments suggesting that men experience
similar situations of abuse and violence as women and need similar
services. Equality of service provision and acknowledgment that
men suffer similar levels of violence and abuse as women appears
to be the central theme of the men's rights movement.

Male practitioners cannot afford to be silent. They need to
engage in the debate on men's services and challenge the emerging
discourse of men as victims (particularly the notion of men as
'victims' of feminism). This is not to suggest that services cannot
be targeted to men. In certain areas programs need to be specifically
for men, such as violence and suicide prevention, and so on.

Some male workers are beginning to take responsibility for
specifically male issues, such as violence. Men Against Sexual Abuse
(MASA) is just one example in which male practitioners are

beginning to work on issues relating to men's domination in patriarchal society (see Pease 1995). It needs to be strongly stated that men in the human services need to take a profeminist stance (see Christie 1998; Pease 1997; Pringle 1998). For male practitioners, taking a profeminist stance is problematic and engages men in examining their own sexist and oppressive practices. This is personally difficult, though it is a demonstration of commitment to a process.

The contradiction for male workers is not to construct the care activity as other than 'emotional labour' (see Camilleri 1996). Emotional labour is necessary and at times an unrecognised component of work. Emotional labour needs to be flexibly organised so that the needs of others can be met. It involves dealing with the difficult emotions of others. It is being able to understand and interpret the emotions and feelings of others. There is a tendency in male-dominated professions to construct the activity in a masculine discourse (see Williams & Thorpe 1992). For social welfare practice, emotional labour provides for an understanding of the 'giving of oneself' within an intimate, personal but not a 'friend' relationship. It is hard work, as emotions have to be handled and space allowed for difficult and fraught emotions.

The language of care needs to be articulated so that the 'invisible' nature of the work can be recovered and displayed as complex and demanding great skill. The assumption embedded in patriarchal society that caring for someone is a natural feminine characteristic needs to be constantly challenged, as men are often 'let off the hook' and not confronted with issues of care.

Men care, and recognition of that is important for men working in the human services. The challenge for men at present is to work closely in partnership with feminists and to be self-reflective. Anti-sexist approaches also need to attend to the cultural, social, economic and political contexts surrounding practice. The links with feminism are important, as practitioners can examine the issues of gender, class and ethnicity as well as the interface between these.

Pease (1997) refers to 'unsettling' men. Male practitioners need to be unsettled. Men both as workers and clients need to rethink the structures and processes in a patriarchal society. Men are part of the 'caring for' activities in the human services. Their stories and narratives of working collaboratively with women colleagues and with both men and women clients are an important aspect of reconstructing care.

CONCLUSION

This chapter has outlined some of the issues facing men who work in the human services. It needs to be recognised within the human services that men are not invisible and are part of the direct service delivery to clients. Male workers have been historically privileged within the human services. There is recognition by many male workers that their practice has to be more transparent and open to scrutiny. There is a concern that male workers have colluded with male clients within family work and child protection. There has been debate regarding the place of men within certain practice areas, in particular the abuse of women and children in care settings (see Christie 1998 and Pringle 1998). This debate, however, should not lead to further separation of women's and men's work in the human services. The issues need to be confronted by male practitioners and safeguards put into place so that women practitioners and clients are not oppressed or exploited.

Gender is so much part of the everyday world that human service work must involve questioning the gendered experiences of both clients and workers. This is not 'easy' practice. Practitioners are overworked in agencies in which resources are scarce and are dealing with clients who are experiencing problematic life situations. It is, however, too easy an option not to question and reflect on gender issues. Male practitioners cannot afford to ignore gender in the workplace. They need to examine themselves in relationship to the reproduction of patriarchal structures and processes and develop practices that are congruent with a pro-feminist position. The practice of human service work is invisible (Pithouse 1987) and we need to make more transparent these practices including gender identities.

Those practitioners who work in caring roles do so in the midst of patriarchal discourses. The challenge for men is to question the assumptions and roles of practitioners. It is also to reflect on their practices and develop strategies that circumvent the reproduction of patriarchal processes. It is unfortunately too common in community service agencies to see oppressive practice by males in which they reinforce stereotypical assumptions of appropriate conduct and roles for men and women. Male workers need to take responsibility for that conduct and question those processes in which the gender order is constantly reproduced.

PART II

GENDER-BASED PRACTICE APPROACHES FOR MEN SEEKING CHANGE

4 | Making connections: Working with males in families

Kerrie James

Despite changes in gender arrangements signalled by women's increased presence in the workforce, women remain the primary carers of children (Horst & Doherty 1995). While traditional gendered arrangements arise in the context of economic and social structures, family and couple therapists are faced with the immediacy of responding to the 'walking wounded'—men, women and children who suffer under traditional patriarchal, gendered hierarchies. In their work with families, therapists are confronted regularly with fathers who are absent or peripheral, mothers who are overburdened and lonely, and children who suffer as a consequence. Fathers who are actively involved in child care, housework and the intimate details of their child's life, elicit considerable interest and wonder!

Over the last decade, health-care professionals have increasingly recognised and expressed concern about the emotional and physical wellbeing of males in our society (Fletcher 1999). Spurred on by the women's movement, some men have begun to examine and challenge traditional ways of being male and the risks entailed in dominant constructions of masculinity (Connell 1995; Pollack 1998; Real 1995). The field of family therapy, having paid considerable attention to changing the position of women in families, is facing the challenge of how to best help men and boys. Family and couple therapists encounter men and boys experiencing relationship breakdown, school failure, violence, substance abuse, depression and the ubiquitous 'attention deficit disorder'. This chapter, in contributing to an increasing focus in family therapy on men in families, argues for an understanding of men which interrogates and challenges the role of traditional masculinity in the interpersonal problems men experience (Deinhart & Myers-Avis 1994; Carr 1998; Real 1995).

In the first section, I examine how traditional masculine identity does not reflect the diversity of men's lives and constrains men's full participation in family life. In the second section, I examine how men's engagement with power impacts on their relationships; and in the third section, I explore attachment and relationship issues in working with male clients. The fourth section addresses difficulties for therapists in engaging men in therapy and the final section overviews some useful interventions to assist men and boys in families.

ISSUES OF IDENTITY: MASCULINITY, EMBODIMENT AND DIVERSITY

Traditional masculinity is part of a binary opposition, which defines maleness in opposition to femaleness. As 'strength', 'endurance', 'rationality', 'dominance' and 'control' are seen as defining attributes of masculinity; 'weakness', 'passivity' and 'emotionality' are seen as defining characteristics of femininity. Male and female socialisation encourages boys and men to be strong, that is, not to be weak or to cry. They are encouraged to be competitive and it is accepted as a sign of successful masculinity to engage in the odd fight, to separate from their mother, and be disparaging towards women. Some have argued that distancing from women and all things feminine is the hallmark of traditional masculinity (Real 1995; Pollack 1998).

Males define and interpret traditional masculinity in different ways. Connell (1995) argues that there are many varieties of masculinity. Men and boys differ according to, for instance, culture, class and sexuality, in how they align themselves with traditional masculinity. However, a mantle of traditional masculinity hangs over most men, particularly those in patriarchal cultures. Therefore, men are faced with decisions about how much they should accept or reject aspects of masculinity. In rejecting aspects of traditional masculinity, men place themselves in a position of embracing qualities that have traditionally been the province of femininity. It is in fact a challenge for a man to integrate these aspects of himself that have traditionally been alienated. Can he bear to embrace anything that is labelled 'feminine', or does it have to be detached from the label? Do women recoil in the same way if they are challenged to embrace masculine attributes? Probably they do, although there seems to be much greater flexibility for women.

Men and women are all constrained by gender norms. But what are the constraints for men and how can therapists help men embrace something within themselves that may defy and challenge the ideal image presented to them by their own fathers? Is it disloyal to embrace what your father could not?

The term 'men's issues' confronts us with a totalising conception of men, as if 'male' is always clearly identifiable, and, as if all such male issues or concerns are the same for all men. The influence of postmodernism has overturned the privileging of gender as the dominant discourse that defines individuals. What has prevailed instead is a more complex intersection of fluid and enduring conceptions of the self, incorporating variables such as culture, race, sexuality and class. This requires therapists to broaden their assessment and intervention strategies when working with men and families in order to consider multiple and conflicting power hierarchies that generate a range of relationship tensions.

I am struck by the variations between men in the degree to which they adhere to aspects of traditional masculinity. For example, heterosexual couples often experience a pattern of relating in which the man is more emotionally distant, and tends to withdraw from his partner who is more likely to be emotionally expressive. This 'distancer–pursuer' pattern is often reversed around sex—the man pursues sexual intimacy and the woman, not feeling emotionally close, withdraws. However, in the following case, the pattern was reversed.

Peter, aged 46, came to therapy distressed about his relationship with his wife Angela who was 38. They had been married for fifteen years and did not have children. Angela had been involved in academic study over the last five years and Peter had experienced her becoming increasingly distant from him. He cried as he faced how rejected he had been feeling and his fear of losing his wife. When seeing both of them, it emerged that Angela had always been somewhat more reserved and distant in the relationship, whereas Peter was more likely to want more closeness. Angela,

on the other hand, had previously pursued Peter for sexual intimacy, but had been losing interest. He was the one who was more
likely to want to talk and work things out.

This case and others challenge the usual assumption that all
men are emotionally less expressive and are less likely to pursue
intimacy. Among men as a group, there is enormous diversity and
our gendered stereotypes of 'masculinity' or 'maleness' often do
not fit a particular man. There are more differences within the
genders than between them (Connell 1995).

I have also learned something about men from working with
women in relationships with each other. In working with lesbian
couples, I am constantly surprised by how similar the couples'
problematic issues and patterns of interactions are to those of
heterosexual couples. Conflicts experienced by lesbians may appear
to reflect traditional gendered patterns, but on closer examination
may have more to do with broader structural influences, such as
employment demands.

Nicola and Jenny were in conflict over their parenting of their baby
daughter. Nicola's demanding job as the senior accountant with
a multinational company resulted in her working long hours
with occasional nights away. Over a year, conflict had escalated
with Jenny feeling abandoned and trapped. The baby showed a
preference for Jenny that meant that Nicola was on the outside
even when she was there.

This situation mirrored the typical concerns of a woman feeling
abandoned by her husband in the demanding world of work. This
shows that what we often attribute to differences between men
and women as arising from socialisation are sometimes the result
of broader socioeconomic structures. These structures, such as
men's capacity to earn high incomes and the nature of jobs or
professions that assume an availability to work a full week or long
hours have a major impact on family relationships. As the lesbian
couple has shown, such demands create a context in which relationship conflict is somewhat inevitable regardless of gender. But
is there any aspect of conflict between men and women that arises
entirely from gender difference? Gender is a fundamental category
that defines individual identity and is embedded in language,
culture and history (Goldner 1991; James 1983). Internalised within
individuals, gender shapes our experience of the world and of the
other. Much of this internalised sense of gender is developed

through our position as either dominant or subordinate within power hierarchies.

THE EMBODIMENT OF POWER

Family therapists are often confronted with the socially sanctioned power men hold over women and children. Dominant discourses encourage therapists and other service providers to help men acknowledge their power in conjunction with acknowledging responsibility for the abuse of this power. How do therapists reconcile some men's experience of powerlessness in their relationships with their higher income, higher status and dominance in the public sphere relative to their female partners?

Males often occupy simultaneously dominant and subordinate positions in Western cultures and are positioned as having more power and status than females. Many men, however, express feelings of powerlessness. They feel they cannot influence their partners or the course of their relationships. Some men also experience powerlessness in relation to their own struggles to get better jobs, to be higher paid, or more successful. Men of colour, Indigenous Australian men, and men from non-dominant cultures may be excluded from sources of power that define successful attainment of masculinity (Boyd-Franklin & Franklin 1999). Similarly, relative to black women, black men are embodied with higher status, but while they may be able to exercise *power over* white women, they have less *status* in relation to white women.

One major reason many men can feel powerless (even though women see them as powerful) is because they harbour a deep insecurity about their 'masculinity'. They are therefore vulnerable to the demands or criticisms of women (and other men) which they interpret to mean that they are viewed as less masculine than the image they so dearly strive to attain and hold on to.

Men's power is embodied; that is, it is located within their physical beings. They hold most of the positions of power and have most of the material wealth compared to women. It also arises from the fact that men are (on the whole) taller and physically stronger than women. This means that, no matter how oppressed or powerless a man is in his relationship, or in the wider society, by virtue of having a male body he is positioned or inscribed in our culture with dominance or higher status, which confers privileges. These attributions of status permeate our cultures and therefore our psyches, and are perhaps what Goldner and others mean when they say that gender is a 'fundamental' category, something so embedded within our psychological and physical selves that we cannot step outside it (Goldner 1991).

It is often difficult for men to appreciate that they cannot shake off the power ascribed to them no more than a leopard can shake off its spots. In fact, men are powerless to divest themselves of power because male dominance is entrenched in our cultural, social and political practices and also in our psyches. Despite this, however, men are capable of recognising their embodied power and of challenging discourses that position them as dominant.

Colour is also a marker of status and 'whiteness' is an embodied characteristic infused with power and status. In most cultures, white people are more privileged than people with dark skins (Dolan-Del Veccio 1999). Therefore, men of colour find themselves simultaneously occupying both dominant and subordinate positions.

When cultural hierarchies ascribe dominant and subordinate status to certain groups, it is important that therapists address the impact of this differential power on relationships. Family therapists need to explore and acknowledge the various power hierarchies existing between themselves and their clients or between partners and family members. This is particularly complex when traditional hierarchies are reversed, for example a male client sees a female therapist, or a black female therapist works with a white male client. One could continue to enlarge on the dominant or subordinate embodied characteristics that pose challenges, contradictions and complexities for therapists, who themselves as therapists occupy a position of status or power in relation to their clients. Managing such complexities between themselves and their male clients presents different challenges for male and female therapists.

ATTACHMENT AND MASCULINITY

Research in the area of attachment provides family and couple therapists with a framework for understanding personal relationships. Attachment theory emphasises the importance of an infant's early secure attachment to a parent in ensuring the infant's psychological and physiological development. Security of attachment continues to be important throughout a child's development.

Fonagy (1997) argues that secure attachment may protect a boy from the negative influence of delinquent peer groups. Recent research has been exploring the nuances of parent–child interaction, taking account of the child's individual temperament. The varying capacity of parents to emotionally attune to their child, and recover from 'misattunements', is an important factor in the child's developing self-concept and ability to securely attach (Stern 1985).

Researchers in the area of gender have revealed that both mothers and fathers respond differently to boys and girls. Mothers are more likely to push boys prematurely towards independence and autonomy (Silverstein & Rashbaum 1994; Chodorow 1978) The father's love is often contingent on his son fulfilling a particular definition of masculinity (Goldner 1995). Both parents may deny the boy child's dependency by withholding comfort when he is upset, encouraging denial of vulnerability. In striving to be assured that boys are sufficiently masculine, parents may override their son's needs for ongoing connection, comfort and affection. As boys are slower to mature physiologically and are more active, parents may be overly punitive or dismissive towards them. If boys receive subtle messages not to cry or are pushed away from mothers by either parent who fears they might create a 'mummy's boy', they begin the process of alienation from their emotional selves that is the hallmark of traditional masculinity (Pollack 1998; Real 1995; Silverstein & Rashbaum 1994).

Consistent misattunement will result in the child developing anxious or avoidant attachment, and negative conceptions of themselves and others. As they show an increase in externalising behaviours and are often more difficult to manage, parents are more likely to resort to physical discipline. This in turn increases the boy's feeling of rage, humiliation and self-hate, which may heighten his resolve as an adult to not let anyone hurt him again. He becomes avoidant, distancing in relationships and prone to becoming violent if his partner separates (Dutton 1995).

Therefore, it is probably not far fetched to hypothesise that traditionally accepted ways of parenting boys create boys who are insecurely attached. Harsh discipline, criticism, lack of warmth and the experience of not having his feelings acknowledged and validated has the effect of creating a boy with a hostile temperament. Most men who have been brutalised in the process of developing masculinity, believe others dislike them, which according to psychoanalysis may originate from the man's own projection of self-criticism onto others. When others do not respond warmly, this man feels victimised, and is prone to violence. Male socialisation, which a boy experiences in other important life contexts such as schools, sport, peers and the popular culture, may only cement his alienation from himself. Any experience of loss, such as parental separation, will create anxiety as intense emotions threaten to emerge, threatening the shaky basis of masculine self-esteem.

As traditional constructions of masculinity and femininity in the context of patriarchal cultures are ubiquitous, issues of gender identity arise in the therapeutic relationship. Male and female therapists are confronted with a range of issues when working with male clients. The following section considers gender issues arising in the relationship between males and their therapist, and the issues for males in utilising couple or family therapy.

THE THERAPEUTIC RELATIONSHIP

Although each gender faces particular challenges, both male and female therapists ought to be able to engage and work with male clients in couple or family therapy. However, engaging men in couple and family therapy is difficult regardless of the gender of the therapist. This is because of both client and therapist factors (Shaw & Beauchamp 1999; O'Brien 1988; Carr 1998). Therapists may feel challenged by men who are reluctant, sceptical or challenging towards the therapist. Such behaviours on the part of a male client can trigger a therapist's anxiety and elicit the therapist's gender-based assumptions about the male client. Such a negative interactional pattern, unless quickly turned around, will inhibit the man's engagement in therapy or lead to poor outcomes. Other factors, such as loss of neutrality or being construed as taking sides, will also compromise the man's ongoing engagement. The therapist has to be able to challenge abusive behaviour or unfair arrangements without losing engagement with either party.

Jones (1995, p. 19) argues:

> Therapists, whether male or female can be aware of the degree to which their own gender premises and prejudices are likely to affect their perception of clients. This awareness makes it possible also to notice premises and prejudices in relation to their own gender.

Awareness of one's own gender reaction is an essential component for effective therapeutic practice. The situation is more complicated when the therapist is a member of the dominant culture, for example a white/Anglo female therapist, who is consulted by a black, Asian or Hispanic male client. While the man's patriarchal values may be the issue for the therapist, the therapist's lack of knowledge of his culture may be the issue for the male client (Lau 1995).

Issues for male therapists working with men

During supervision and training, male therapists often experience complex feelings when working with male clients. While having the advantage of being able to empathise with and understand their male clients, they are not immune to feeling threatened or frightened by a man's anger or competitiveness. The male therapist may avoid confronting their male clients or collude with them out of identification or fear of conflict. There is also a tendency for male therapists to be threatened by intimacy with male clients, and to move towards an intellectual and rational way of functioning (Isparo 1986).

In working with couples and families, male therapists must manage their own counter-transference reactions to men and women in relationships. They may project onto the female client their own experience with their wives or mothers, or vestiges of patriarchal or misogynist attitudes and side with the man. Likewise they may project onto men unresolved issues with fathers, teachers or other men and consequently side with the woman.

Male therapists also have to manage their own reactions to either male or female clients who put them on a pedestal, ascribing the therapist the role of expert as a male and as a therapist (Morgan 1992). Male therapists, by being aware of their embodied status and power, and their consequent ability to influence clients, can use this to empower others, by recognising and validating their client's strengths and capabilities. They are in a good position to assist male clients to acknowledge dependency needs, develop their awareness of emotions and change inequities in their relationships with women.

Issues for female therapists working with men

Female therapists face a range of challenges in working with male clients. The female therapist and male client combination may embody aspects of traditional power arrangements between men and women, and if not dealt with, the therapeutic project may suffer. Male clients may be dismissive towards their female therapist, or believe she lacks credibility or authority by virtue of her gender or age. This is especially the case in relation to men from more patriarchal cultures (Lau 1995). Female therapists themselves may struggle to feel empowered with some male clients, especially those who behave in an abusive or controlling manner.

Some of these difficulties may be understood as resulting from the confusion of two opposing and competing hierarchical relationships: the man is simultaneously higher in status than the female therapist by virtue of being a male, and lower in status by virtue of being the client. Similarly, the female therapist is positioned as one up in the hierarchy as the therapist, but one down as the female. In couple and family therapy, the presence of the man's female partner will further complicate the hierarchy, in that he could now feel excluded from a real or imagined coalition between the women.

Consequently, the female therapist needs to be aware of the impact on a man of being positioned as both a client, and as a client of a female therapist. In couple or family therapy, the therapist needs to maintain balance in exploring and understanding both clients' perspectives, and seek to understand the man's perspective, crossing the gender difference. Having awareness of one's own gender issues or blind spots, and an understanding of gender as a social construction that does not entirely capture any of us, the female therapist may be able to work successfully with men, even those who are abusive, contemptuous or emotionally disengaged from themselves and others.

If a female therapist has herself felt disappointed or let down in her own relationships with her father, partner or son, she may be rejecting or angry towards a male client, whom she believes is behaving similarly towards the women in his life. On the other hand, some female therapists may side with the man and be more critical of women. A male client's transference issues, for example, seeking to dominate his female therapist or falling in love with her, can both be viewed as the man's fear of vulnerability, dependency or losing control (Morgan 1992).

In summary, male and female therapists face different challenges in their work with male clients, particularly in couple and family therapy. These challenges arise from embedded and embodied power dynamics that pose particular counter-transference problems for a therapist.

Therapeutic issues for men

Men are less likely than women to initiate couple or family therapy, and are more likely than women to drop out once they start (Shaw

& Beauchamp 1999). This ought not to deter the therapist from actively connecting with husbands and fathers and seeking to engage them in the work. Engaging the father in family therapy and facilitating the father's active participation is predictive of better outcomes (Carr 1998).

In order to maintain a man's engagement in therapy, therapists need to develop a 'fit' with each man. This may require the therapist to focus on solutions, behaviour change and direct advice that many men seem to prefer. One study has shown that interpretations, reframing and the use of metaphor are popular interventions with men (Dienhart & Myers-Avis 1994). Taggart, however, questions the usefulness of cognitive approaches to working with men that are based on the belief that men are more rational, cognitive or intellectual. He believes that some therapists shy away from facilitating men's affective expression, fearing that men cannot tolerate their emotions. Taggart suggests that the men he sees want to, and need to, experience their pain (Taggart 1992).

The interventions that therapists use need to take account of these nuances in the therapeutic relationship. The following section identifies a range of interventions that are useful for working with men in couple and family therapy.

THERAPEUTIC INTERVENTIONS WITH MALES IN FAMILIES

The interventions that are outlined in this section address the issues raised by the problems posed by traditional masculinity, embodied power and insecure attachments attendant upon traditional masculinity.

Challenging traditional masculinity

Although a large majority of men may present as if they are in control, rational and only needing advice or a solution, therapists need to assume that men do experience a range of emotions. In response to relationship conflict, some men experience extreme degrees of anxiety, which may or may not be revealed to their partners. Feelings of fear of loss, weakness, vulnerability and hurt often cause internal turmoil because they threaten the man's view of himself as a man.

A man may wish to avoid awareness and expression of those feelings at all costs. He may fear being humiliated, being seen as a failure or being abandoned or punished. Many men do experience relief, however, when their inner world of feelings is acknowledged or brought forth by the therapist. Partners may also respond positively when they are invited into the man's inner world of vulnerability.

Therapists can approach a man's distress by exploring the pattern between the man and his partner or his child. In family therapy, this may be conflict between parents about the father's controlling or authoritarian parenting style, where the mother is viewed by the father as too 'soft'. In couple therapy, it may be conflict about a man's distancing or the woman's pursuing behaviour. Exploring the inner world of the man's thoughts and feelings in relation to his behaviour in the relationship begins to deconstruct, or tease apart, the traditional edifice of masculinity.

> Peter and Angy came to therapy because they were arguing about their three young children and how to raise them. Peter criticised Angy for being too soft, pandering to the children's wishes and not setting limits. Angy was concerned that Peter intimidated and threatened the children, was 'over the top' in how he reacted to minor misdemeanors. An underlying issue was Peter's work in the armed forces, which meant he was away a lot of the time. Upon returning, he felt excluded from the much closer relationship his wife had with their children. The therapist explored what it was like for Peter emotionally when he came home. He expressed feeling hurt and rejected, unable to emotionally connect, incompetent and unloved as a parent. As Angy had experienced Peter as distant and quick to anger, she felt surprise and relief to know of his inner feelings of vulnerability. The therapist prescribed a 'welcome home' ritual, and worked with Peter on developing a 'softer' more nurturing relationship with his children.

Confronting self-harm

Therapists can challenge traditional aspects of masculinity that are obviously harmful to the man or his family, for example: working long hours; neglecting his health; over use of addictive substances; expressions of anger to the exclusion of other affects such as hurt or sadness; domination and control of others and self-righteousness. Depression and attachment anxieties may underlie contemptuous, controlling or aggressive behaviours and need to be addressed if other family members are to be protected. Exploring the man's relationship with his own parents can shed light on his current experience of fathering or being a partner.

In the above case, it emerged that Peter had not been close to his own father who had been abusive to him and his mother, and, from adolescence, had taken on the role of supporting and protecting his mother. He had erected an emotional wall in order not to be hurt by his father's emotional abuse. He hid his fears from both his parents, his father because of his abuse, and his mother because of her vulnerability. The therapist drew a connection between his current defensive style in relation to Angy and to his experience of having to protect himself from his parents. The therapist was able to use Peter's experience with his own father to encourage him to soften his approach to his children. In this instance, the parents agreed to the therapist's suggestion that the mother should manage the discipline and the father should concentrate on learning to relate to the children.

Exploring aspects of masculine identity

Therapists need to create a space for and validate a man's individual story of his history and experience of masculinity in relation to class, race or sexuality. Therapists can assist men to identify the impact of experiencing violence, racism or homophobia on their own self-worth and in relation to their own subsequent oppression of their female partners, children or others.

There are a number of areas of men's lives that therapists can assist men to change when they are no longer effective. In the following example, the therapist explores the meaning of work and career after a husband has been made redundant.

A married couple with two teenage children came to therapy because of the husband's depression. Two months previously he had been made redundant after working as a manager for twelve years. The therapist discovered that both of them had believed that the husband should work fulltime to support the family, and had done so for 21 years of their marriage. Although Julie was now willing to get work, it was the prospect of her working that distressed Roger the most. It emerged that he had grown up in poverty and it was a sign of his success as a man that he had been able to support his wife and family. After exploring and validating the meaning of work for both of them, the therapist was able to challenge him to accept that his wife's contributing to the family's income did not have to reflect on his adequacy as a man. Roger found part-time work and was able to enjoy spending more time with his children.

Dealing with unfairness

It is often helpful for therapists to be able to assist a couple to understand that conflicts arising from the division of labour about housework and responsibility for child care may reflect the traditional patterns for men and women in the wider culture. Usually a woman is more likely to feel that these arrangements are unfair resulting in her emotional withdrawal and anger towards her partner (Knudson-Martin & Mahoney 1999).

It is important that therapists working with couples and families are able to identify inequities in relationships and intervene to ensure that unresolved resentments are expressed and resolved; resentments that lie dormant, usually fester unnoticed, until finally, the injured party announces they want to end the relationship, begins to have an affair, or abuses a child (MacKinnon 1998).

Exploring power, dominance and subordination

Therapists need to be skilled in identifying abuses of power, including physical, verbal and sexual abuse towards partners and children. If men in families are benefiting from positions of dominance, they will not be inclined to relinquish privileges unless their partners insist on change. Sometimes the only way to help men change is to help women to not tolerate abuse or exploitation and use a form of leverage to obtain change. This may involve obtaining legal intervention and/or leaving the relationship. Some men will change rather than lose the relationship, and at this point a therapist can be helpful in assisting the man to take responsibility and make reparation (MacKinnon 1998; Goldner 1991).

Exploring attachments

By exploring family of origin relationships, a therapist can help a man be aware of the source of his fears of rejection or loss, and facilitate him to respond more appropriately to his partner or children. In return, they will respond more positively to him, resulting in increased security in the relationship with them. Insecurely attached men who pursue their partners for increased closeness, can be helped to 'self-soothe' rather than harass or intrude on their partners (Schnarch 1997). Avoidantly attached men can be helped to express their thoughts and feelings rather than distance or 'stonewall' (Gottman 1994).

In the following case, a therapist intervened to help a man deal with conflict he experienced with his new partner.

> Ian revealed to his therapist painful childhood events, which included his mother leaving the family when he was eight. He and his younger sister were then sent to live with his aunt. Although Ian recalled this as a difficult time, he did not show any trace of distress in recounting the experience.
>
> A few sessions later, he and his partner Liz had an argument in which she had blamed him for something which he felt was very unfair. In a flash of rage he pushed her, resulting in Liz falling down some stairs and twisting her ankle. In unpacking this incident with the therapist later, Ian stated that he had felt overwhelmed with rage and feelings of pain. He connected the feelings of anger he felt towards Liz with his feelings of anger and hurt he felt when his mother abandoned him. This time he could not but feel the pain.

By 'unpacking' violence, therapists often uncover painful rejections or losses that have not been acknowledged or expressed and which need to be worked through (Goldner 1991).

One of the benefits of working with families in therapy, is that parents can be assisted to understand their son's emotional needs and reassured that nurturing, emotionality and expressions of vulnerability are not signs that their son is failing or that there is something wrong with him (James 1999). In challenging the tenets of traditional masculinity in child-rearing, therapists can facilitate both parents to emotionally 'attune' to their son. Stern has described 'attunement' as the parent's immediate mirroring, recognition and validation of the child's affective expression (Stern 1985). Through observation of the father or mother interacting with their son in a family therapy session, therapists can assist parents to mirror, recognise and validate.

> Michael, a boy aged fifteen, came with his single-parent mother to family therapy because he had seemed depressed, and had refused to go to school since his girlfriend broke off their relationship. Michael's mother, Nancy, was extremely worried that Michael had inherited his father's depression, which was a factor in his untimely death from alcohol a few years earlier. During the session,

the therapist asked the mother to talk to Michael about her concerns. In observing the interaction the therapist noticed that Nancy very quickly started to tell Michael that he had to forget this girl and get back into his study. The therapist assisted the mother to 'hold' on this line of advice, and to just listen to her son, repeating back what he was saying, validating his feelings without offering advice or suggestions. In a short while Michael had explored his feelings with his mother acting as therapist and both of them could see that his grief and depression was appropriate to the situation of losing his girlfriend. The therapist encouraged the mother to continue to attune in this way to facilitate his expression of grief. The mother needed support to do this, as it triggered her own unresolved loss in relation to her husband and losses from her childhood.

Although the therapist had not mentioned gender or masculinity, she was still able to challenge one of the most significant tenets of traditional masculinity, which problematises boys' feeling as not masculine or not normal.

CONCLUSION

This chapter has presented a framework that explores how masculine identity, power and attachment impact on men's and boys' experience of themselves in family relationships. It outlines how a family or couple therapist might approach some of these issues in working with the problems presented by men and boys in families.

Men represent a diverse group of sexualities, cultures, religion, races and classes and individual men differ in their 'take up' of traditional masculinity. However, power hierarchies within each of these dimensions mean that men are most often, but not always, constituted in discourse as 'subjects', with 'others' who are subordinate. Some men, however, are positioned as subordinates or as 'others' in hierarchies where other men, and sometimes women, are dominant.

Professionals therefore face a range of intersecting and complex issues when they engage and work with fathers, husbands and sons in a therapy or counselling context, including their own positioning as classed, cultured and gendered subjects. Therapists must elucidate the power dimensions of family relationships and address them in their work with men in families.

An attachment framework recognises the emotional and relational needs of men and their fear of showing such needs. It problematises 'masculinity', which depends upon the disavowal of such needs. A man's fear of and aversion to anything that can be vaguely construed as 'feminine' means he acts to deny or disown significant experiences and continues to position women and children as the repositories of such affects, that is, to position them as 'other'. The implications for his relationships with significant others are profound. Therapists, however, may be reluctant to challenge a man's adherence to traditional masculinity, through fear of losing engagement with him. Sometimes therapists are so complicit with traditional masculinity themselves, that they collude and protect men, rather than challenge what they fear is a man's fragile sense of himself.

The ways in which discourses of masculinity interfere with attachment and become enshrined in the personal lives of men and their relationships is the essence of family therapy.

5 | Neither colluding nor colliding: Practical ideas for engaging men

Mark Furlong

In this chapter I will set out practical ideas about engaging men in a casework relationship. This discussion will proceed in three steps. Initially a brief review of the principles of engagement will be offered emphasising the importance of neither 'colluding' nor 'colliding'. A second level of engagement-related thinking will then be considered: how to identify, and work with, the language, symbols and metaphor that 'this man' you are working with can understand. A third level of thinking will offer material about the importance of, and some practical ideas for, being able to influence the dynamics of the casework relationship by differentially positioning oneself in order that the contact is neither an arm wrestle nor a pseudo-mutual hug. Several case examples will be used to illustrate these ideas. Prior to introducing this material, the following may help the reader situate the three steps.

Much of the available practice-oriented material that, for example, explores case management or cognitive behavioural therapy, speaks as if an expert unilaterally undertakes procedures upon, 'does it' to, a passive, unreflective other rather than talking in a language that articulates beginnings and middle phases of participation and the question of what kind of relationship type is desired. With respect to the desired type of relationship between service users and practitioners in the human services, the aesthetic and practical goal of engendering partnership and collaboration appeals.

Partnerships are about participation and, at their best, have a synergy, an energising 'togetherness' in pursuit of a shared goal or a sense of making a joint journey. Partnership and collaboration are about having a very practical dream about the nature of the project and this is not an idle fantasy but an everyday ambition designed to promote the prospects for cooperation. In saying this it should be clear that good partnership and collaboration are not based on sameness and foggy agreements. Rather, they are based on difference in role and expertise and in perspective and contribution.

The traditional professional assumes: 'I am the expert so, if you agree with me, you are cooperative, have insight and are compliant; if you see it differently, if you disagree, you are resistant, uncooperative and are non-compliant'. This, of course, raises the reality of power and its differentials. Such dimensions need to be named so that 'who writes the rules and who owns the game' is explicit. Establishing—let alone maintaining—collaboration and partnership is often difficult, perhaps even like trying to play Scrabble without vowels, yet however difficult it might be, the question is: Is there a better alternative? Is it better to be involved in arm wrestles, to be the boss, to be the clinician?

ARE MEN A DIFFERENT SPECIES?

There is a risk involved in even the most pro-social of generalisations. For instance, against 'accepted' definitions men do tend to be less emotionally and interpersonally literate but, as Weingarten (1991) observed, there is a danger in assuming that a particular definition of intimacy is the only one or, more generally, that one form of subjectivity is superior (Mens-Verhulst 1993). The notion that either gender has dominion over particular emotional, relational or conceptual competencies seems neither attractive nor useful: 'the claim of innate female superiority in regard to women's capacity to nurture, their empathy and intuition, and their rich emotional life, is as counter to the egalitarian spirit of feminism as the claim of innate male independence and rationality' (Hare-Mustin & Marecek 1986, p. 209). Despite statements that can 'truthfully' be made on the basis of verified probability, one should be reticent to grant these generalisations as universal. So, given that guardedness is required, what might usefully be said in relation to engaging men?

In general, one engages men as one engages 'people', that is, the engagement phase involves observing a number of principles: it is not about attempting to change the other but about establishing respective roles and responsibilities; it is about clarifying, often in terms of complex more or less overt negotiations, the purpose and structure of the work and so on. Thus, in so far as it is possible to distinguish phases, engagement is about 'setting the stage' for the change-oriented work that is expected to take place later. Engagement is concerned with trying to entrain a process that, over time, will set up the client as their own expert. Fundamental to this is 'to start where the client is' (Goldstein 1983). The following case vignette introduces a theme that is central in relation to beginning work with men.

Case vignette

Vic was a large man who had an intense if not intimidating presence. Although not imposing in actual size, Rita, his partner, was also striking with a tungsten voice and 'I've seen it all and I'm not scared of anything' gaze. Along with my co-worker, I'd first met them, with their very large and high energy family, in the agency waiting room where we both worked.

The family had been referred to our centre by their local child protection service because of extreme and apparently escalating difficulties with two of their teenage children. Although it eventually became clear the parents were very perturbed by, and were feeling powerless about, the difficulties with the two older children, they were not about to bow from the ankles to any professional or procedure. Amongst a host of factors inclining them towards scepticism and (at least) gruffness, they had been told by the Children's Court they had 'to attend counselling as directed'.

This first meeting was a tense affair. At times my co-worker and I were stood over, abused and at the very least not heard. At times I felt frightened by Vic's physicality, weak in the presence of the intensity of Rita's uncompromising 'you've got to take life on its own terms' attitude and more than a little invisible as a person as I was being spoken to as if I was a soulless representative of a brutish social order.

Reflection

What I remember acutely feeling during this session was an uneasiness that I might be colluding with, or might already have colluded with, what was just plain wrong. This is always a risk when trying to engage, and stay engaged with, any individual from a 'different side of the tracks', to lean a little too far their way in order to be seen to be on-side (as there is an arguably greater invitation to collude with those who are ostensibly of the same cut as you). One can and should make one's position clear but one does not wish to be discourteous by overtly disagreeing or dismissing the views of the other even if this seems necessary for pro-social and ideologically sound reasons. Overtly disagreeing or dismissing their views risks colliding with the other and results in a different kind of engagement problem to that of collusion. Finding a balance, a net effect, that neither colludes nor collides is the golden mean sought by all human service practitioners and sometimes this feels like trying to square a circle.

For example, many middle-class practitioners allow themselves to be painted into a pallid dispensability by non-psychologically minded 'window shoppers' who want practical assistance rather than insight or an apparently non-pragmatic and timeless contemplation of feelings or the past (Mayer & Timms 1969). All too aware of this danger we were clear we had a responsibility to the parents and the children not to be precious and to remain committed to respecting this family's cultural, aesthetic and ethical realities however different they were to ours.

We wanted to maximise our chances of forming a partnership with the parents but, at least from time to time, it felt like we were on different sides in a values battle and collaboration in times of war is wrong. For example, this family's culture was that the children—both girls and boys—lived in an unfair and nasty world where being able to both take and administer violence was a skill to be practised and valued. Given violence was an everyday part of family and neighbourhood life, where did that leave my co-worker and I? Could we collaborate with this belief?

The connotations of the term 'collaboration' are generally held to be positive: we wish to collaborate with the families we work with as we wish to collaborate with 'colleagues' in the broader service network. Yet, the term collaboration is one of those interesting words, exactly like its cousin-term 'resistance', with a particular, context-specific meaning. In times of war if one actively and willingly cooperates with the enemy, one is pejoratively labelled a 'collaborator' and collaboration in such circumstances is a crime just as to 'resist', and be a part of the 'resistance', is a positive imperative (Furlong 1996). It can feel like a binary, like one of those really unhelpful either/or situations: 'Can you run with the fox *and* with the hounds?'

Viewed from the opposite direction it seems that it can be an advantage to be a practitioner who is not of the same age and class as your clients. It seems that there are occasions when, for example, there are opportunities if one is *not* of the same sex or culture as one's clients. An assumed sameness between clients and practitioners can inject a perceived disloyalty when differences are expressed. Certainly, initial engagement seems less problematic but later it can become 'sticky'. In these situations I sometimes feel constrained by assumptions of affiliation.

WHY IS THERE THIS TENSION BETWEEN 'COLLUDING' AND 'COLLIDING'?

Although experienced in a variety of ways, men from many cultures and ethnic backgrounds tend to share a sensitivity to the question of public presentation; that is, there appears to be a cluster of phenomenologically-related states, such as embarrassment and shame and the danger of 'losing face', that together speak to the notion that men have a particularly configured, and possibly skittish, 'social self' (Longres 1995). This notion is consistent with, but has not previously been correlated with, the poststructural premise that identity—both male and female—is ongoingly evolving, is multi-sited and is contextual, for example, as in Buchbinder's (1994) idea that male selfhood has a 'conferred' quality and in that sense is dynamically constituted, rather than monadic and timeless. If it can be publicly conferred, it can be publicly disqualified; if identity is performative, it is a 'state' characteristic not a 'trait' quality.

This is consistent with the premise that male identity and selfhood, like that of women, is 'relational,' as well as 'autonomous' (Guisinger & Blatt 1994; Paterson 1996). Thus, in some 'telling' situations one useful generalisation is that men may be particularly sensitive to maintaining their sense of dignity and social status because this sustains their sense of self. It may be important not to inadvertently threaten a male's fragile sense of self by being sensitive to the risks involved when men exhibit feeling states, correlated with 'loss of face' and 'shame'.

In so far as this fragility is characteristic of men, men tend towards 'colliding' so as to have a sense of 'identity as difference'.

Collision defies dissolution by firming personal boundaries. Rather than risking this dynamic, workers can act in a manner that does not directly threaten the conditions of male selfhood (aware that the opposite risk is also present, that is to 'collude' in order to avoid the male's anger or rejection). The following sub-section explores a common speech pattern among males which may help set the stage for being able to 'start where the client is'.

MEN'S TALK: LOWERING THE REGISTER RATHER THAN INCREASING THE PITCH

While it is often assumed that good work with men has to attend to the matter of the males' suppressed feelings (Egan 1997; Miller 1983), less confronting and more subtle approaches may be helpful. Mindful of approaches identified with the narrative therapy tradition (White & Epstein 1989; White 1992), the following will focus on the more limited question of 'men's talk'. For example, the language habits of the typical Anglo-male tend to have a characteristic signature. Unlike what the average practitioner is exposed to, if one talks with men from the country and the trades one finds a language that is, in the first instance, spare and minimal. One hears a vernacular of particular economy and of regular, at times even elegant—although not always observed—circumlocution. If a man encounters someone who is abrasive or even confronting, the sure-footed man will say, but say without a backward step, to the other: 'go easy'; if bad luck strikes, even if this risks a long established desire: 'yes, it was pretty ordinary'; if disaster strikes: 'I guess we are struggling a bit'.

Of its essence, the ANZAC stare is stoical: understatement is thought to be characteristic of what is well mannered and manly. Whatever one's view on the appropriateness of 'male speak' it is fair to note that this language practice tends to lead to the filleting, or at least the radical coding, of the emotional from accounts of experience and the self. This habit is consistent with valuing of steadiness and persistence. In this way the 'hysterical', the dangerously capricious, the emotional, are projected out and disowned. Emotions or, more precisely, being emotional is that which is unstable and therefore unsafe. In a direct parallel to the West's denigration and yet romanticising of the 'mysterious' East (Said 1968), male stream culture does an 'us and them' on that which is emotional: the realm of the emotional is both dangerous, as it risks one's self-control, and yet mystified as it is sacred and not to be touched except in special circumstances.

Thus, it is regarded as legitimate for all men to become occasionally emotional. For example, sporting heroes are allowed to be emotional—when they kiss their baggy green cap on reaching their ton—and the common man can also, within very particular circumstances such as the death of an intimate, be emotional. Yet this specificity of legitimation is both so extremely circumscribed, and the character of the expression so overripe, that this condition acts to generally de-legitimate expressions of feeling. Without a powerful legitimation, being emotional falls clunkily beyond the high walled pale.

Additionally, a complex thread that accompanies this language practice is the male's habit of being both semantically and inter-actionally, albeit playfully, provocative and concurrently ironic. While the valorising of understatement and the phlegmatic is arguably a characteristic of male stream cultures, Australian men often have a particular facility with, and share a particular intimacy around, what might be described as a kind of tempered, even disowned, provocation in language practices and social interaction: if you like someone enough, or if you wish to test their claim to membership of the group, you will 'stir' them. This is often expressed, as things generally are, with the use of irony and of linguistic opposites: redheads are called 'bluey'; and what do you call an Australian cricketer who is famous for scoring slowly— 'Slasher'; what do you call an English cricketer who is famous for scoring slowly—'Barnacle'. It is a delicately nuanced matter ensuring that irony is not blurred with sarcasm, playfulness with mockery and there is often an edge, a potentially serrated quality that voids intimacy, if the implicit is named or explained. At times this code can be so embedded as to have its actors captured by the game; at other times the quality of invention and intimacy is so assured as to be both racy and validating.

This language pattern both reflects current men's modes and also prescribes how the emotional and the inter-personal will be performed. Yes, this pattern can be problematic but it also reflects a value system that is both embedded and, in many ways, is admirable. For this reason the language habits are representative of 'the way it is' and need to be worked with. Moreover, to say these practices are very gendered is a truism yet they also represent a broad trans-gendered cultural practice that has class-based and broadly distributed historical roots: many Australian women, and not just working-class women, act—and represent themselves—within the conventions and possibilities of this linguistic pattern and value system.

Practice implications

If one is an outsider, such as a professional, these language habits need to be respected. Broadly, practitioners should try to work within, even as they may try to subvert (Goldner 1992), the males' language code mindful that this code is one that speaks of values as well as preferred forms of speaking. In so doing one is often called to do the opposite of what is recommended by the imperial texts of counselling psychology that stress the centrality of feelings and their expression—generally act in ways that lower the emotional register rather than increase the emotional pitch. Do not prescribe grief, for example. The preferred pattern language for talking with men does not involve being emotional about the emotional; one can be direct about it—but not directly emotional—as the emotional is a sacred exception rather than the everyday feature. Practitioners can be intimate with male service users but in a men's way.

For example, if something awful has happened, like when the farmer's last dam ran dry or the year's crop got washed away, as mentioned above, and the cocky dryly notes that this is a 'pretty ordinary' state of affairs, it follows that a professional asking the man to 'grieve' might just find themselves not taken too seriously. One might choose to respond sparely, perhaps metaphorically, in this situation—we can both know what we are talking about, that we are talking about feelings, without rubbing the man's nose in it, without risking personal boundaries or causing shame. In cross-gender situations perhaps particular care is required.

Some useful approaches are:

- to be spare and understated;
- to be prepared to be playful: you can 'stir' as long as it is not understood as mocking or confrontational;
- monitor one's language in order to avoid language patterns that alienate; for example, avoid coming across as 'wussie' or too serious and be sure to disavow counsellor-type buzz words, for example, the word 'issue' as in 'the issue here is . . .';
- often men are more comfortable with a language of action to understand that ('we can meet to plan/reflect/(even) do' rather than 'we can meet so that you can share your feelings'); and

- as long as it is not patronising and feels comfortable to the worker, to speak positively into the language habits of the other, via the particular, for example, via the other's occupation, or the more general and often the more gendered topic of sport.

Being careful about your metaphors: Not becoming captured by the game

Returning to the practice world, the father of a six-year-old spent some time in a first interview loudly complaining that his daughter was consistently not doing as she was told. This man was not just annoyed and disappointed, he also in some sense seemed shamed by the daughter's behaviour as he understood it to mean that she was not just disobedient but uncaring. When asked if he sometimes thought of her as 'young' rather than 'bad,' he said, 'Of course I do'. The worker then said, as a kind of throwaway, 'Yeah, I guess tadpoles can't jump' and moved the conversation on without labouring the point.

One does not need to be Erasmus to know that the way a behaviour is understood is crucial to how one responds and this is the theme Goldstein (1983) examined in his perennially relevant paper 'Starting where the client is'. This chapter argues that workers can and should attempt to elicit data on the 'lived experience' (Schutz 1972) of the other in terms of how this experience is understood, how it is interpreted, rather than act as if reality is unambiguous and consensual. This theme has almost certainly been prominent in the practice wisdom of social work for a hundred years, has been published and explicitly discussed since Mary Richmond's principle text (1917) and has been described in terms of 'the client's own story' for very nearly 50 years (Hamilton 1940, pp. 51–2).

In so far as a metaphor is perceived to provide a successful fit with the circumstance in question, it can make a reasonably effective claim to relevance if not outright dominion. If this claim is also supported by a set of resonances rich in lived experience, such a fit is radically potentiated and our metaphor is transformed into incontestable simile. Rather than the map being seen as a relatively good representation of the ground being surveyed, it can now almost literally become substituted for that territory. Thus the power—and the danger—of using embedded, and therefore implicit, metaphors such as those from the sporting world. Not only do these culture bearers have an active face validity in terms of being seen to represent salient facts relative to our, using the sports example, 'hard but fair' current socioeconomic world, they can be employed, both constructively and disingenuously, to draw from the collective resonance associated with all the sports that each one of us has participated in, with our pride in our current and past sporting heroes, with the populist image of sports, and so on. Thus, caution, as well as creativity, is in order.

For example, in the late 1980s I was having a first session with a young man and his family where the adolescent was having persistent difficulties at school and at home. In my view his father, who was a career officer in the services, appeared to be caught up in an unhelpful dynamic where the more the son withdrew and sniped the more the father lectured and berated. As is almost inevitable in such circumstances, this drew the other parent into the position of defending her son which, as one should expect, further polarised the parents' respective positions and, in turn, embedded the problematic dynamic. Rather than being able to either just 'hold' (in the psycho-dynamic sense) the tension of this situation or, less likely to be helpful, being able to non-blamingly comment on the pattern, I used the deliberate re-frame: 'I think your son is running point for the family'.

Clearly, the use of such an explicitly military, and therefore emotionally loaded, metaphor was highly inappropriate *especially in a first meeting*. It was blaming, disrespectful and—is there a better word to use—*smart arse*. In first contacts we have to be courteous, we are trying to build relationships. Thus, given how powerful metaphor can be it is essential to be not just sensitive but accountable in the metaphors we choose to use (Lowe 1990; Furlong 1997). This is especially true when the metaphor is the more powerful for its embedded and therefore potentially insidious effectiveness.

POSITIONING: THINKING ABOUT HOW WE ACT IN RELATION TO, RATHER THAN ACT UPON, THE OTHER

The notion of 'positioning' has been discussed in the exchanges that generate and sustain the profession's practice wisdom yet there is little published literature specifically on the topic (Real 1990) even if there is a more extensive literature on adjacent themes, such as alignment (Selvini-Palazzoli *et al.* 1980), neutrality (Cecchin

& Lane 1993) and in poststructural theory (Davies & Harre 1990). There is also considerable material available based on a sophisticated understanding of the importance of positioning even if the notion is not elaborated per se, for example, Anderson and Goolishian's (1988) idea of refusing to be the expert by taking a 'not-knowing' stance; Jenkin's (1990) work on 'invitations' to responsibility; reflecting teams (Young *et al.* 1989) and, in general, much that lives within the narrative tradition.

These authors tend to prescribe that practitioners appear unaligned and non-directive as this contributes to a collaborative, change-oriented dynamic. Thus, 'it is thought to be more effective if practitioners position themselves to be seen as expert in relation to knowledge without being seen to be instructive in relation to people' (Furlong & Lipp 1995, p. 113) although there is the occasional exception (Silver 1991). That is, it is thought to be more engaging to avoid a language of hierarchy, not to tell people what to do or what they have done wrong.

So far I have begged the question: what is 'positioning'? Defining this notion is difficult and can perhaps best be approached obliquely. You are driving your car along a windy, hilly country road when you begin to catch up with a slower vehicle. If your intention is to set yourself up to most easily pass this car, is it better to be close behind or should you leave a gap, a considerable space, so you can accelerate and overtake when a chance arises? How is it best to 'position' yourself? What are the likely consequences of tucking yourself right behind the other car; might this set you up to miss chances and to become frustrated and blaming in relation to the other driver?

To understand the notion of positioning one must leave the traditional modernist, expert role set where the professional is presumed to be objective, to be meta to, the client to whom this lofty impartial expert is in the business of neutrally dispensing truth deposits. Rather, one can understand that the professional and the client are respectively located within a set of contexts not least of which is the dynamic, the dance, of their specific interaction. Thus, from a constructivist perspective the worker is understood to be 'positioned' within, rather than outside of and able to act neutrally and instrumentally upon, the client.

If one accepts that it is neither possible nor desirable to act procedurally as if the other is inert, the converse is that one needs to be reflexively aware that in doing and saying, that is, by taking position X (given it is understood that the term 'position' is a rubric term), this doing or saying is an active step in the process of defining a dance. That is, I need to be aware that what I do and say is simultaneously both an act of self-expression, a truth claim and is at the same time an interactional communication, a signal about the kind of relationship and the kind of process that is to be enacted. One needs to be aware that the other responds to—dances—in part because of their interpretation of the information received from what we say and do.

Thus, taking positions—for example, being optimistic that this client you are now talking to will be able to change—can tend to prompt a dynamic which, in turn, may establish a pattern in the here and now within which participants either tend to 'dig in' or 'move on', to defend or 'unfold'. If the repeated sequence of the client–worker interaction is: the more I say to you 'you can change', the more you feel convinced you are not being heard, then the inadvertent consequence might be that (despite the semantic message being 'you can do it') the dynamic, the process, that is enacted is such that the other gets more embedded in asserting 'No, I cannot do it any better!'. This is the territory Bateson (1973) discusses in terms of 'symmetrical' and 'complementary' patterns.

It is understood across a range of approaches that one cannot unilaterally change the other. The use of positioning is based on this premise and, if this premise is respected, it follows that in order to work towards change, one endeavours to engage the other in a dance that 'brings forth' the new, rather than re-invents the old. If I act differently, if my step or stance changes in my contact with you, this may change the dance. At one level the notion of positioning relates to the question of 'alignment': are you aligned with the mother, the daughter, or the referrer, etc? The notion of alignment and positioning is also about more abstract qualities: are you aligned with—or against—the prospects for change?; are you aligned with the 'emotional' or the 'pragmatic' with respect to your tones of voice and linguistic pattern?; are you aligned with— or at an angle to—'tightness' or 'openness' re body language? For example, if one is a woman, and one is seen in the typical counsellor stance, how might the following be interpreted by this man?; leaning forward, being ripely attentive and serious, nodding the head, saying 'I hear what you are saying and the issue here is . . .' Is it positioned to be experienced as engaging, as an open invitation to talk within a mutually defined space, or as a signal that the practitioner owns the game and writes the rules?

Case example

Darren was a nineteen-year-old man who had been, with his family, referred by his case manager to a family support centre six months after he had returned home from twelve months in a slow stream rehabilitation program. This residential program had assisted Darren to improve, but not completely remove, a set of behavioural and cognitive deficits that followed a motor bike accident.

At the time of the accident Darren had been a second year apprentice with an interest in motor sports and heavy metal music who, at that time, had been engaged to Rita. Since the accident, but not necessarily because of the accident, Darren and Rita had separated, he had become unemployed, was viewed by his parents and his case manager as a 'quite likely' suicide risk, was sometimes hostile to his younger siblings and parents (with whom he lived), was regularly using large quantities of cannabis, had lost his driving licence and had, in general, become socially withdrawn. His rehabilitation assessments were clear: he had sustained a significant frontal injury and could not be expected to lose his discernible motor and cognitive deficits.

Although seemingly less than enthused at being brought along by his mother to talk, Darren appeared to be both forthright and frighteningly distant at this first meeting. He said he thought his life was 'stuffed' and that 'nobody, and this includes you', can make any difference. He spoke with an apparently clear understanding of his deficits and it seemed the only time he became interested was when he said there was no point in meeting again.

Commentary

How should the practitioner position her/himself to maximise the chance of engaging Darren? One knows Darren will not ask for help: 'Yippee, I would really like to talk to some middle-class stranger about how I am an inferior, embarrassing shadow of the person I once was'. Expecting this kind of 'insight' is like expecting Darren to enjoy having his nose rubbed in it, like expecting him to want to stare at the sun through a telescope.

As mentioned earlier, the modern approach is to position oneself in a neutral way, as wanting to be seen as offering an invitation to Darren. In this way one avoids the (odious) scent of hierarchy and instruction and, of course, there are many reasons for thinking this approach has much to offer in many, if not most, situations. Yet, although this approach often has real advantages, in working with a number of young men in Darren's kind of situation it seemed that unless it was 'performed' with some show, some theatre, it lacks enough edge to engage with the only energy Darren displayed: his defiance. Perhaps, it might be more useful to not give him a choice mindful there is no risk-free option. Perhaps the greatest constraint to engaging Darren is his sense of hopelessness. Maybe, to bluff Darren into coming along is more likely to be face saving for him: 'I guess I better go, I'll get more grief for not showing than for turning up'. Such bluffs may backfire but also may get him along and if this happens this at least gives the worker a chance.

CONCLUSION

One's positioning is enacted in the conscious and non-conscious expressions or the positions one takes in terms of the many dimensions involved in one's use of self: behavioural performance, semantic content, affective tone, attitude, personal style and so forth. When viewed from this perspective one is—each human is—of necessity, a 'performing self' and the question is: how can I monitor and modify this performance in the service of my role and goal?

The topic, like what has been said earlier of metaphor and language, probably sounds at least unaesthetic if not downright amoral: how could it be said that our work is the same as that of a car salesperson or the politician—how can I sell this car, how can I look convincing kissing this baby? This talk of acting done by performing selves is presumably the common language of those business training programs devoted to improving selling skills.

Working therapeutically with people is, among other lively matters, always something of a conundrum. As in games of romance, where the eagerness of one party comes to be associated with unattractiveness while the coolness of the other positions this one towards desirability, therapists can too obviously seek what they think is best for their clients. Clearly, it does not always work this way but it happens often and powerfully enough to be worthy of consideration. One does not have to agree with Murphy, that exemplary existential character, when he says 'love requited is a short circuit' (Beckett 1936) to have an understanding of the often odd and poignant nature of human dynamics.

6 | Working with men's defences against vulnerability

Mal McCouat

The purpose of this chapter is to outline an approach to working with men developed in a specific context of private practice. The framework is primarily psychodynamic, and is informed by critical theory and feminism. The chapter outlines the theoretical framework and examples of its practical expression, followed by an appraisal of its strengths and weaknesses.

The emphasis I place on vulnerability grows out of my personal experience, as well as my clinical practice and academic work. Both my natural father and my first stepfather were casualties of the Second World War. My father was killed serving in the Royal Air Force and my first stepfather died when I was seventeen. As my mother's oldest son, I learned early about her need for me to help her to feel better, to be good, to achieve, and to regard her as a perfect mother. I also learned that men, while God-like, were also absent, and that my own separateness and gender could easily be brought into question by feelings of obligation. These learnings shaped my professional life, from early experience in the Probation Service to 30 years' teaching social work.

THEORETICAL FRAMEWORK

Masterson (1988) has developed an approach which, though not aimed specifically at men, is useful because of the central importance of what he calls the 'abandonment depression'. For him a group of painful feelings (anger, loss, helplessness, hopelessness) attended a lack of support afforded the vulnerable, fledgling self during early life. Support is also necessary for consciously experiencing these feelings, so in the face of its lack they are avoided and the young person sets up a defensive 'false self' based on the demands of the environment. Later contexts calling for activation of the self initiate the danger of being abandoned again, and the 'false self' defence is brought into play, 'acting out' the feelings rather than experiencing them consciously: activation of the self leads to anxiety which leads to defence. Implicit in this is the recognition that, since the unconscious idea is to avoid the pain of abandonment, activation of a defensive self will always involve exploitation of the self and/or of other(s) in some form, as a method of survival. If the complementarities of this exploitation begin to break down or seem threatened, larger defences and more extreme exploitations and acting out are called for.

At the societal level, Peggy Reeves Sanday (1981) investigated the contexts of primarily pre-literate societies in relation to their patterns of gender relationships. She found that those societies which were more stressed by shortages of food and/or forced migrations, and/or war and conflict were more likely to have a 'segregated' pattern of gender relations characterised by greater male power and privilege. She wondered whether this power was taken and accorded as compensation for the socially defined greater dangers involved in male activities in these externally threatening contexts, again as a matter of survival. Conversely, she found that where societies were not, or only a little, stressed in any of these ways, gender relations tended to be more respectful, more equal, and roles more shared or overlapping. Various methodological difficulties attended Sanday's research, but anthropological data from Gilmore (1990) and Levinson (1989) support its general thrust. Work on the patriarchal development of Mesopotamian civilisation by Lerner (1986) also refers to its very harsh context.

The framework I bring to my work combines these two perspectives. A systemic pattern of gender exploitation constructs men with a public capacity and legitimacy to defend themselves against the danger of consciously experiencing their own vulnerability. They exploit and draw collective and individual sustenance from the vulnerability of others: women, children, some other men, older people, physically less able people, etc. This defensive pattern has a structural face in that patriarchal processes locate men there with the power and sanction to do this, and a personal face in an individual lack of awareness of ordinary human feelings and experiences of vulnerability. Men's consciousness is split: public power, private and unconscious vulnerability. The public face is held in place by acting out the vulnerability, making the other experience it so that defensive and material benefit accrue to the more powerful position. It is a defining feature of power asymmetries that this can 'successfully' be done; it is a defining feature of ideology that it is made to appear natural.

My work with men is usually aimed at helping them to become more conscious of their experience of vulnerability in whatever form it takes in their lives and relationships and to manage it with more conscious decisions, using it to reach out realistically for support and as a base for compassion for and acceptance of themselves and others. Accompanying this is working towards their recognition of the effects on others of acting out their vulnerability defensively, becoming as aware as possible of what it might feel like to experience being with them in whatever context is relevant. This means becoming accustomed to acting in the outside world with simultaneous consciousness of vulnerability, rather than cutting this consciousness off. Being clear that the usual contexts of organisations, work and sport are, in various degrees, hostile to this consciousness, or even abusive of it, can form the basis for critique of, and opposition to, their offending and exploitive characteristics.

In a segregated gendered context in which men control language, logic, meanings, boundary making/keeping and decision-making, it is no wonder that the giving and taking of support has been identified as 'female', while the former are identified as 'male', structuring in men a split between their sexuality and their emotional needs. More especially so since the structure of economics and gender mould the family in highly subtle, basically non-verbal patterns placing male partners/fathers more distant from children, and female partners/mothers closer to children and traditionally more dependent on them both emotionally and for vicarious self-expression in the public sphere. Chodorow (1978) has given a similar account and her perspectives are useful here.

For boys, this means a highly ambivalent relationship with the original vulnerability that is the experience of every human child, being nurtured and protected by the parent of the other gender and being aware of her power to withhold this or not be able to give it to abandon. At the same time there will very often be a mostly implicit sense in which the boy's morality, lovingness and success are felt by him to be expected by his mother, even needed by her—a load that sometimes shows up in the defensiveness that we express when questioned or challenged, especially by female partners. Combined with the more distant and powerful expectations for performance of fathers and the competitiveness and violence of male contexts, this produces extensive vulnerability, very difficult to live with consciously and survive. It makes sense that the latter would be labelled 'female', and be denigrated publicly and repressed privately and be the object of shame if begun to be experienced explicitly.

It seems logical also that we should charge our female partners with looking after our more vulnerable selves without open acknowledgment that we are doing so. That they often comply (though this is becoming less common), owes much to their own complementary early training in being aware of, and responsible for, the needs of others. Our sense of entitlement in this cues us to feel immense fear, shame and failure under conditions of abandonment—precisely the feelings we try so hard to get away from by means of a structural power/personal defence. On the other hand, if we as men were to acknowledge the degree to which we need support, we would value and acknowledge, both personally and structurally, the immense giving, generosity, and the sheer hardness of the work of being attentive to the needs of others, the work that we capitalise on, gain strength from, and take for granted and denigrate—the work, mainly done by women, that silently and implicitly undergirds and repairs the destructive effects and processes of the patriarchal system.

In this situation, a sense of abandonment is easily evoked, not only by separation of a major kind, but also, and more problematically, by the withdrawal of support implied and expressed in criticism, challenge or the expressing of need in some form by the other person, because here we are required to stand with our own personal resources, and sometimes to put those resources at the service of empathy for the other. The commonness of problems of relationships of all kinds shows how difficult it is for men to do this—indeed, how few truly personal resources we have.

MIRRORING

One of the ways all this is expressed interactionally is in what may be called a gendered collective and individual need for mirroring.

Seidler (1989), Pease (1997) and Connell (1987) have written about the way men are authorised to speak not only for themselves but also for others, and Masterson (1988) has described the individual defence of a narcissistic mirroring requirement. At both levels, the process involved tends to cancel out any responses other than those that 'go along with' the story that the speaker is developing. Institutionalised violence in its many forms, and the ordinary political process can be understood in this way. Individual men often respond with legalism, discounting, deprecation, rejection, impatience/anger/rage, disdain, scorn, overriding, fear, shock, hurt, truculence, evasion, etc so as to secure a mirroring response to the maximum extent possible. The effect is to cancel out the individuality and separateness of the other. On the surface, this would seem to bespeak a high degree of self-sufficiency, but this is only an appearance. The speaker can only gain an insecure foothold on his own sense of self so long as it is buttressed and reproduced by the self-effacement of the other in being drawn into more or less total fusion with the speaker's words, meanings, feelings and actions. The listener's power is undercut.

The patriarchal prescription for heterosexual couple relationships is: men speak and act, women mirror. It is not surprising then that so many contemporary relationships, having started out this way, strike problems under the contradiction built into it: that the very thing depended upon and denied, the nurturing of the woman, rests long-term on her capacity to be a fully expressive self. When the latter begins to happen, the lack of reciprocity becomes clear, and explicit conflict and change in some form starts to happen.

The way this often presents itself in the context in which I work, is that the female partner expresses pain about not being supported, acknowledged, or about betrayal or violence in some form. At some point the male partner may be persuaded to join the consultation. Alternatively, less often, the male partner is the one who makes contact expressing fear, confusion and doubt about threats by his partner to leave, or a range of responses from suicidal depression to rage and threatening murder concerning an actual separation.

The typical way in which this situation expresses itself is in the man's conveying pain about having 'fallen out of love' with his partner or experiencing being trapped indecisively between two or more women. Voyeurism or child sexual abuse are reasonably common. Sometimes the female partner complains of her partner's being unable to make decisions or take responsibility, or senses a lack of commitment. If she moves on, the desolation of the man can be very difficult for him to survive. While it may often seem on the surface that he is a victim, the exploitation of the life force of the other is obvious at a deeper level.

In both forms of the need for mirroring, I have developed a set of procedures that are both verbal and non-verbal. I mirror physical posture and follow the other's gestures. I anticipate the endings of sentences and apologise profusely if the anticipation is wrong. I echo the last few words of statements, perhaps slightly accenting the emphasis that he himself employs. Although this subjugates my own expression of myself, the deliberateness of doing it offsets the effect. I also use this to get an early tentative idea of how much vulnerability is defended—the more subjugation of myself required the more defence is likely to be needed, the more caution indicated and the more serious the situation.

The aim, though, is different in relation to these two forms of defensive need. In the situation where the person is directly reproducing himself, mirroring builds a platform of safety so the counsellor can try to be heard as a voice, benign through mirroring, though also dangerously alien. In the more vicarious expression of the need, on the other hand, it is important to be careful about interfering with what comes from the other person, in case he subjugates himself to the idealised words of the counsellor.

In the first context, I find myself frequently saying towards the end of the early sessions, things like: 'I've been listening carefully to you for the last 50 minutes, and I wonder if it might be possible for you to hear me say some things as briefly as I can'. I then give a summary of what he has said as if I am an advocate for it, sometimes giving some emphasis to elements in which he seems to feel misunderstood or badly done by. Then I say to the effect: 'I think you're likely to find what I'm going to say difficult to hear, very difficult to accept, but I need to say it to be fair to you', and I then make some suggestion about how he might have had to learn to expect so much of himself and everyone, to control things so much etc. to help him to cope with difficult situations/feelings that he's forgotten about, and this may make it hard for other people around him to feel acknowledged, heard or appreciated. I then congratulate him and thank him for listening to me because I realise 'listening is pretty hard sometimes'. 'This capacity to listen that I've just experienced tells me that you have the courage to receive difficult things as well as to survive.' If he goes along with all this, the beginning basis is laid for exploring the elements of it further.

With the other version of the need for mirroring, I mostly find myself prefacing what I say with variants of 'Don't take too much notice of this, it might be only me', or 'This is just an idea', etc., or discussing the danger that, at exactly the point where he seems to be asking for direction, I might actually give it, and that would be terrible because it would prevent him from grappling with the vulnerability involved in speaking and deciding for himself.

Where I know that physical violence or sexual abuse is occurring, I follow this up directly, keeping the need for mirroring in mind; not sidestepping the issue is the first consideration because doing so would subvert the integrity of the work and compromise safety. The abuse must stop as a first priority.

INTERRUPTING 'ACTING OUT'

This intervention involves 'catching' the first feelings before acting out and 'holding' them. This work opens up opportunities to reframe the context of masculinity and to explore the 'then' in the 'now'. Using the above as a base, suppose the other person says something like: 'I don't know what came over me, I just got so angry' or 'I just found myself looking through the window at this woman getting undressed' or 'She's so bloody messy, food stuffed in the fridge, clothes lying around, no good with money' or 'Why does she always criticise me, find fault with me?'. An examination of what preceded these experiences can provide something of a short cut to the world of self-exploration and can be quite pivotal to the whole work.

Some current context (criticism, frustration, stress, etc.) threatens to require the person to re-experience some forms of vulnerability: abandonment, loss, sadness, fragmentation, uncertainty, fear, insecurity, feeling overwhelmed, dying, drowning, falling, etc. Instead of consciously experiencing them, the person acts out the experience, transforming it in the process, for example, from fear to rage, or from sadness to depression, or humiliation to scorn and self-perfection, or uncertainty to control. This process interactionally attempts to externalise the avoided experience and place it in the experience of someone else. It has been Masterson's (1988) particular contribution to point out how this happens, not only in a generalised way, but in the very minute particulars of ordinary living. It happens moment by moment in the space of seconds. An implication is that if the person can gain access to an intimation of the avoided experience that he/she flashes across in a milli-second, the wellspring of the defensive pattern can be grasped as it happens; potentially then a realm of possible awareness and expansion of options for decision and responsibility opens up with far more immediacy than merely exploring generally the early experiences of the person's history.

A parallel way of saying this is to note what has been long known: that in compulsive acting out, the addictive behaviour needs to stop before underlying feelings and problems become available. Again seeing this in minute occurrences of ordinary concrete situations forms a potential entry point. So I will say: 'Take yourself back to when that happened. Remember as precisely as you can when she said/did that. Now, what's the very first feeling you felt, or actually didn't feel, immediately?'. Usually the response is a bemused repetition of what he had earlier reported—'anger, etc.'. But if one perseveres: 'No, just before that', he will edge closer to something else—'tightness', 'tension', 'here we go again', 'feeling blamed', and then perhaps, 'shamed', 'powerless', 'guilty', 'sad', or similar. Sometimes it is useful to give the theory first: giving a cognitive framework fits how men often approach things. Role playing the situation can also help.

Then it is possible gradually to encourage him to explore other situations where he feels the same, to suggest that he hold on to the feeling rather than change it into something less vulnerable and less useful; to find his own suitable words for it, to become an expert on when he is more or less likely to feel different strengths of it, etc.

It also becomes possible to suggest that he allow the feelings to take him back to contexts and similar experiences earlier in his life and explore how the defence arose and why it was needed. This begins to shift the emphasis from failings that the current people in his life seem to be forcing painfully on him, to those caretakers whose responsibility it was to provide a safe context for the acknowledgment and understanding of vulnerability and pain. Who the 'real enemy' was becomes clearer, and it is possible to suggest that what happens in the present is often in the nature of a trigger: if there is no ammunition, there is merely a click—a response more or less in keeping with the stimulus. When the gun is loaded, however, meanings/feelings and actions are overburdened by the past—individual and collective history. That combination becomes the real enemy.

It is possible to introduce here the idea that the specific framework for boys makes acting out vulnerability, rather than consciously experiencing it, the preferred, the male, the gendered, option, with painful consequences for those seen as more vulnerable than ourselves, particularly girls and women, and also some men. The experience of too much danger which also means too little support together with the collective tidal wave of narratives about what constitutes maleness marginalise compassion for the vulnerability of the self and for others. A useful alternative frame to offer is one based on a new form of male courage. Rather than the 'over the trenches' kind, a new form of courage could be enacted by men refusing to reproduce what has been given to them by their childhood/society/history, by carrying their pain and vulnerability, by paying the price themselves, and turning away from the inner and outer invitations to pass it on, as a re-production of the tradition would have it; instead to stand by oneself and others who feel vulnerable, and encourage them to express their pain; this will sometimes mean taking responsibility for hurtful things we have done or are doing.

A variation of the above procedure is to imagine the difficult context without the acting out option. 'Imagine you're in X situation, and then imagine that it is just not possible in any way, the option simply doesn't exist, to be angry, violent, sexual or whatever, imagine that the option you took is totally blocked off. Now, what feelings happen as you face that?'

Another suggestion is blocking the acting out response, and looking inwards to see what happens. This is particularly appropriate with the more obviously compulsive addictions, but can be useful with violence etc. as well: 'When you feel like doing X (for example, stalking a separated partner), set yourself just once not to do it, and see what comes up for you immediately, when you don't. Observe what makes it difficult to stay in that place.'

It will be clear already that if the painful feelings were not difficult to bear, they could be borne; when the man is beginning to experience his feelings without defence, he will often feel intolerably vulnerable, shameful and guilty. There may be a real risk of suicide or violence. So it is very important that the man avail himself of, or re-vitalise, networks of support (for example, a group for men) particularly during this period. I also usually make myself available on call during this time.

MOURNING, REPAIRING AND RECONSTRUCTING

Much of the working through of all this involves two sources of grieving. One relates to renouncing needs for childhood forms of support and acknowledgment that once were entitlements as a natural part of growing up, but which now in adulthood are not appropriate in that form; they cannot now be made up for directly. A double renunciation is necessary: for then, and for now. Almost unlimited sadness is appropriate, rather than the cutting off which underlays the skilful learning of defensive capacities.

The second is about grieving for a defensive system which served the person well, in that it enabled him to survive perhaps unsurvivable and traumatic situations, and even to flourish in the relevant defensive context. 'Ah,' we say, 'that seemed great though I now know it wasn't really.' A related dimension involves the recognition of time wasted, and pain unnecessarily experienced and caused. 'If only I knew then what I now know,' we say. 'If only I could go back and re-do things.'

The impulse to go back tends to be very strong where the person is struggling with feelings of shame and guilt and the need to be perfect. Less shame and guilt make it more possible for the person to move on. Sources of shame need to be a specific focus, and the person needs to externalise the shame in focusing on the characteristics of the persecuting environment rather than on his own characteristics in order to shift attention away from the latter. It is important for him to remind himself about the myriad ways in which he does and has expressed characteristics different from those shamefully identified by the eyes of others. It can also be useful to clarify that a guilty response is almost never about caring for the feelings of others; it is instead about focusing on one's own needs to feel better, and so interactionally is demanding.

Finding a different locus for sexuality, one based on closeness and vulnerability rather than on physical need, competition and control, often becomes a focus. In the interim it can seem that the work is undermining a sense of sexuality. It can be useful to explain that this is only because men have learned to split sexuality from their emotional life. Since they remain sexual beings, when they have integrated defended against parts of themselves, their sexuality will integrate itself with them instead of with the defences. Similarly work and other forms of self-expression may change focus.

Repairing the hurts of others is prepared for by the preceding work. Essentially it involves listening, on the other's terms, taking on board their perceptions and feelings, and being there while doing so. It is about facilitating them repairing themselves. It also involves doing whatever is necessary to be done, but not in a way calculated to wipe out the hurt. It means that the relationship at this point will be more important than one's own feelings, and that for a time the latter are put on hold, and the focus is on the needs and self-expression of the other. Carrying the pain of regret, remorse and self-doubt is necessary and very difficult. Being unable to repair can be particularly painful.

The kind of help needed here is to respect and acknowledge the courage and wisdom involved, to recognise the pain and aloneness and stand with the man in facing it as a natural and real consequence of his own behaviour, to encourage him not to ask for forgiveness but to listen instead, to remind him that the process is more important than the content, and to recognise that at the time of his hurtful actions, however bad in retrospect, he was still doing only what he knew at that point. He cannot undo it, but what he can do is listen and encourage the self-expression of the other.

USES AND LIMITATIONS OF THE APPROACH

The specificities of the context of its development need to be noted. It is not tested in cross-cultural settings, and applies primarily to work with adults; limited exposure with young men suggests usefulness. A fair verbal capacity helps; intellectual impairment reduces its relevance. A relatively stable environment is an advantage. Most of my clients are middle class.

This chapter sets out a suggested structure that can be used to inform couple work, workshops, training and group work. It reads as if it is about long-term work, but actually most of my individual work is relatively short term, and different male clients are at different points in relation to what has been written here. One of its advantages is that it helps me locate where the person is and what likely next steps may need to happen. It also helps, I think, for a male client to have a sense of what the overall picture is. In a cognitive sense, it makes for a little more safety and certainty; uncertainty is a difficult state for most men. People are so varied, though, that the structure cannot be a prescription.

CONCLUSION

Western cultural history legitimises men in defensively acting out through others their own unconscious pain and vulnerability. This is part of the same process as the historical creation of dangerous environments which keep the vulnerability unconscious. This legacy needs to be changed by the collective construction of peaceful, safe contexts, so far as this is possible in the real world. This is an important frontier for male culture and for humankind. Individually, to develop the capacity, and the safe networks that are required to foster it, to carry vulnerability and pain consciously and responsibly, and to encourage those in vulnerable positions to express themselves and to listen to them when they do, defines the new face of courage for men. The refusal to re-produce pain that is handed down to us—to pay the price ourselves rather than pass it on—enacts that courage in changing both our intimate relationships and that history.

7 | Working with males who have experienced childhood sexual abuse

Patrick O'Leary

> I always thought it only ever happened to me, but lately I had a sense I was not the only man. No one ever asked and I never thought I'd be able to tell. I never forgot about it or the shame.[1]

This chapter aims to introduce human service professionals to theoretical concepts that guide practice responses to males who have experienced childhood sexual abuse. Central to these considerations is the visibility of survivors' experiences and knowledge. The chapter outlines practice responses based on men's own stories obtained through research interviews and practice experience. Emphasis is placed on the sociopolitical and cultural factors that contribute to the adversity experienced by males who have experienced childhood sexual abuse. Finally, exploration is made about possible contributions that human service organisations can make to facilitate proactive service delivery and community awareness of male sexual victimisation.

The challenge for human service professionals who come into contact with males who have experienced childhood sexual abuse is to create a context where their masculine character is not placed under scrutiny or question. Most frequently sexual violence is a male crime with a female victim. This, combined with gender and sexual stereotypes, has largely constructed sexual vulnerability as a feminine trait. When sexual violence occurs against males it can place their masculine character under scrutiny.

The effect of hegemonic masculinity[2] often leaves men isolated with the burden of carrying the effects of trauma caused by another person's violent and abusive actions. Hegemonic masculinity promotes certain ways of manhood that have greater power and influence (Connell 1995). These characteristics and practices include physical strength and active heterosexuality as legitimate masculine traits. Experiences of sexual abuse for males can often be constructed as contrary to these stereotypes of masculinity. As a result, men can feel restrained from speaking about experiences of sexual abuse, because of an awareness of the scrutiny that can occur if they disclose. Isolation in this struggle can result in men exceptionalising themselves as 'freaks' and constructing themselves as to blame for the sexual abuse. Professionals have a role to explore with men their preferred ways of being that may have been obscured by the effect of childhood sexual abuse.

Understanding the history of how child sexual abuse came to be recognised as a social problem of significant proportions is important, so that practice approaches can be clear in their principles and values. This can help professionals to position and acknowledge that men's experiences of childhood sexual abuse occur in a gendered and a heterosexual-dominant culture.

SOCIAL INQUIRY INTO MALE VICTIMS OF CHILD SEXUAL ASSAULT

While men overwhelmingly perpetrate sexual violence,[3] it is not a crime that has exclusively female victims. Vulnerability to sexual violence exists throughout the lifecycle for females; however, males are most at risk in childhood and adolescence.[4] The occurrence of sexual violence against males has been acknowledged more recently, mainly as a result of the greater community acknowledgment of sexual violence against females. It is important to note that this change in community attitudes, albeit not without opposition,[5] has mainly occurred as a result of the political work and advocacy of the women's movement. As part of the process of this social change, researchers have made greater attempts to identify the prevalence and impact of childhood sexual abuse. This research has primarily assisted women activists to demonstrate the legitimacy of their concerns about the often hidden occurrence of child sexual abuse. It is within this body of research that the prevalence of male victims of childhood sexual abuse far exceeded initial expectations.[6]

Estimates into the prevalence of sexual abuse against males vary greatly. Reviews of prevalence research have estimated that a rate of between 2.5 per cent to 36.9 per cent of males and 6.8 per cent to 53.5 per cent of females have been subjected to childhood sexual abuse (Dhaliwal et al. 1996). The large divergence in prevalence rates is often due to different definitions of sexual abuse and sampling methods (Cermak & Molidor 1996, p. 387). An Australian study showed a prevalence rate of 19 per cent of males and 45 per cent of females (Goldman & Padayachi 1997, p. 494). From this information it can be said that prevalence rates of childhood sexual abuse against males are by no means minor.

The increasing awareness of sexual abuse in our community has resulted in an increase in demand for support services. Human service practitioners have largely filled this demand. While the major proportion of the population seeking to address the impact of childhood sexual abuse are women, the number of men seeking assistance is increasing (Swift 1998). A phone-in for reports of sexual assault in the Australian state of Victoria found that 15 per cent of those calling about experiences of childhood sexual abuse were men (Centre Against Sexual Assault 1998).

Increasingly social problems such as mental illness and crime have been linked to past experiences of childhood sexual abuse. Psychiatric populations of men and women report higher than normal rates of past experiences of child sexual abuse (Calam et al. 1998; Read 1998). A study by Fondacaro, Holt and Powell (1999) found that 40.4 per cent of male prison inmates reported being subjected to sexual abuse under the age of eighteen years. Inmates reporting childhood sexual abuse also showed a higher incidence of psychiatric related disorders. There have been numerous studies (Romano & DeLuca 1997; Ryan et al. 1996; Briggs et al. 1994) linking sexual offending to past experiences of sexual victimisation. The aetiology of sexual offending is complex (Briggs 1995). Factors apart from prior sexual victimisation have been linked to sexual offending. For example, Skuse et al. (1998) found that sexual offending was more closely linked to witnessing intrafamilial violence. Many male victims themselves fear that they will go on to perpetrate sexual violence even though they do not necessarily report actually committing such offences (Mendel 1995). Research by CASA (1998) indicated that 21 per cent of male survivors fear that they might sexually offend.

EFFECTS OF CHILDHOOD SEXUAL ABUSE

Many of the overall emotional effects of childhood sexual abuse reported by males and females carry similar labels, such as depression, anxiety and confusion (Heath et al. 1996; Rosen & Martin 1996). However, the gender difference is more likely to occur in the way meaning is attached to these terms (Hunter et al. 1992). Much of the research into the effects of childhood sexual abuse has focused on women. Therefore, many of the results cannot be confidently generalised to men who have experienced childhood sexual abuse. Gender differences in the severity of effects of childhood sexual abuse have been a source of debate among researchers (Chandy et al. 1996). While the debate on severity may continue, many dozens of practitioners consulting with men and women will attest that the effects are more than often impoverishing. The degrees to which these effects play themselves out in people's lives vary, and many factors contribute to these differences. Some research suggests that later psychological functioning is predicted by the severity or characteristics of sexual abuse (Heath et al. 1996). While Sigmon et al. (1996) suggest that social support is an important factor in later coping and adjustment, my experience as a practitioner has indicated that a combination of factors determine the intensity of effects experienced by men.

The effects of childhood sexual abuse on men have been identified by a number of writers. Many of the effects can be classified into Finkelhor and Browne's (1985) four traumagenic dynamics: stigmatisation; betrayal; traumatic sexualisation; and powerlessness. Within these dynamics Mendel (1995) identified three recurring issues for male survivors of childhood sexual abuse: dissonance between the male role expectation and the experience of victimisation; shame and gender shame; and identification with the perpetrator and fear of continuing the cycle of abuse. Three similar themes have been identified by Gill and Tutty (1999, p. 23): society's refusal to accept the reality that men can be victims of sexual abuse; an impaired ability to form intimate relationships; and an impaired ability to form satisfying sexual relationships. Research interviews[7] I have conducted with twenty men who experienced childhood sexual abuse identified four major themes:

feeling stigmatised as a man because of the abuse; blaming oneself for the abuse; confusion; and suspicion of others.

The way in which professionals identify and respond to men who are experiencing these effects can be helped by understanding some of the restraints that can make it difficult for men to speak about experiences of sexual abuse. These restraints often centre on issues that relate to: isolation; shame; fear of perpetrating; and homophobia. Once men have found a way to come forward about experiences of sexual abuse it is important that their story be acknowledged. This may require that the adversity that the abuse has caused be named in a context so that exploration can be made about what it has taken for them to cope. This process can take time so that the effects and coping strategies can be better understood. It is from this type of conversation that professionals can help men reclaim their hope and appreciate their resilience. The remainder of this chapter now examines values, principles and approaches that I have found helpful in facilitating this process.

PRACTICE CONSIDERATIONS FOR WORKING WITH THE EFFECTS OF CHILDHOOD SEXUAL ABUSE ON MALES

Human service professionals have a central role in facilitating a hopeful process that will help men to separate from the effects of childhood sexual abuse. This involves offering individual support and fostering greater community awareness.

Before exploring practice approaches it is essential that the value orientation of the approach be explicit. The particular value positions that I believe to be important include:

- That the experience and knowledge of survivors of sexual abuse inform practice approaches. This is best expressed by Alcoff and Gray's (1993, p. 282) proposal: 'We need to transform arrangements of speaking to create spaces where survivors are authorised to be both witnesses and experts, both reporters of experience and theorists of experience'.
- That approaches be accountable and responsive to structural inequalities that exist between diverse groups (Tamesee & Walgrave 1994). These groups may include differences in gender, sexuality and culture. As Connell (1995) states there is no single masculinity and as such there are diverse groups of men with varying structural inequalities.

It is paramount that practitioners have an appreciation of the difficulties that males may face when they speak about sexual victimisation. The following practice considerations[8] are designed to prepare professionals to comprehend the difficulties that men can face when dealing with the impact of childhood sexual abuse.

Isolation, shame and disclosure

Well, it's just keeping a secret, not letting anybody into your past. You're so frightened basically of what your family might say against you, or scared of reliving the past, that you don't want to bring it up. I had what happened in the back of my mind all of the time, but it felt like if I don't say anything to anybody, well one day I might just end it. And if I went to my grave no one else would ever know what happened to me.

Part of the primary difficulty at both an individual and cultural level about male childhood sexual abuse is the difficulty of speaking about the issue. The issue is not often mentioned in the community. It is thought by many researchers that males are largely under-represented in clinical populations seeking assistance for the impact of sexual abuse (Holmes *et al.* 1997). Adding to these difficulties is men's general reluctance to utilise health and community services (Pease 1997, p. 37). My doctoral research[9] has found that males and females were no less likely to tell someone at the time of the abuse. However, men took significantly longer than women did to speak to someone about experiences of childhood sexual abuse. Most men took over ten years to discuss the abuse, whereas most women took under ten years to discuss the abuse with somebody.

Men who have experienced childhood sexual abuse often experience a complex range of reactions. They often fear other people's responses. This fear is often connected to perceptions of vulnerability, homophobia and misinformation about victims becoming perpetrators. These factors can make certain environments unsafe for disclosures of sexual abuse. Consequently, the decision not to disclose can often be an exercise of good judgment and self-protection.

Professionals in a variety of fields of practice may be in situations where men may take the opportunity to disclose. This often occurs in human service organisations that do not specifically deal with sexual assault. Disclosure for many men has occurred at a time when the issues they are facing are intensely serious and they feel out of control (O'Leary 1998, p. 25). Often significant others play a part in helping men to come forward about sexual abuse. In my practice experience, this has often been a woman to whom the man is close, such as his mother or partner. One man who experienced childhood sexual abuse described how a number of problems mounted after years of being silent about the sexual abuse:

> It was last August when it just went bang! I had sort of handled things up to that stage. I thought things would never change. I must have fucked it up bad. Lost my licence . . . because I got pissed and stoned all the time and did whatever I wanted to do . . . I went with this chick . . . we'd been in the sack together and I had visions of when I was a kid—went back there and it freaked me out. It was after that I got pissed. I was popping Valium too at the time, and ran amuck. Went home on a Saturday and didn't wake up til Monday! My old lady found me on the floor, and I ended up in hospital for a couple of days. That's when I thought I'd better sort out this shit once and for all.

The experience of childhood sexual abuse contributes to isolation from mainstream men's culture. For men to be aware the occurrence of sexual violence against males is by no means a rare occurrence can help to relieve their feelings of isolation. It is also important to acknowledge that, when men disclose experiences of childhood sexual abuse, they are making a stand against two possible impoverishing influences on their lives. First, they are making a statement against the effects of abuse. This is a first step in separating from the abuse. Second, by disclosing and seeking assistance to address the effects of sexual abuse they are making a stand against some of the less helpful stereotypes of manhood, such as men should not ask for help.

Male victims become perpetrators

> I heard some statistic on the TV that 50 to 60 per cent of people that are molested, can end up doing it to other children in later life. This made my worst fears come to life, because I know how what happened to me affected me, and I couldn't bear doing that to another child. I didn't want that.

The connection between sexual victimisation and subsequent sexual offending is often portrayed in the community with simple causal explanations. The fact that the majority of men who have experienced childhood sexual abuse do not become sex offenders is rarely publicised (O'Leary 1998). These media constructions as well as anxiety and confusion can lead to men having fears that they will perpetrate sexual violence. One man explained that when disturbing or confusing thoughts about experiences of childhood sexual abuse are spoken about it requires a response that is respectful and empathic:

> Yeah, the only way I've known to deal with it is to isolate myself, to keep away from people. Suicide one minute, go and have a big cry the next minute, and keep on dealing with the emotions that are coming up and shame that's coming up inside me. I'm on my own with visual pictures that come up, that I might not normally talk about . . . that I'd isolate myself . . . or I'd think because I'm a man and I'm not supposed to be that way, or you might feel bad about me if I actually say that I have a feeling of sticking my hand down someone's pants, stuff like that—I keep to myself because I don't want you to know about that, but then that just keeps on promoting things. I talk about that and get a neutral response from the person who's listening, or overwhelming empathy with what I'm talking of. That's when the healing takes place, and I can let go of it because there's someone in front of me who's not condemning me. This is a new moment.

This quote highlights the context of how the impact of sexual abuse is influenced by many complexities that place particular importance on the response of the listener. The response of the practitioner needs to be emphatic in recognising confusion and shame, as well as being clear that abuse is wrong and irresponsible. It can be helpful to identify that the man's fear of perpetrating abuse is often a stand against abusive ways, and therefore representative of what the man may be wanting for his life, that is, a life committed to respectful and responsible ways of being.

Homophobia

> The whole homophobic thing became fairly important to me. Not that I would have used those words then, but that there was something wrong with me fundamentally as a man, and that I needed to prove my manhood, my masculinity in some way.

Homophobia has a pervasive influence on males, especially during adolescence. Societal sanction against same-sex attraction and partnerships occurs in both overt and covert ways. The institution of homophobic reactions in dominant male culture can create sexual confusion for males who have experienced sexual abuse (Gill & Tutty 1997). This confusion can also lead to secrecy and shame, as well as feelings of inadequacy about masculinity. It is within this context that complexities may arise. These complexities may obscure the power dynamics that are inherent in all acts of abuse. For example, caught up with the influence of homophobia is the idea that if a male experiences sexual abuse from a man, this will somehow mean that he is gay.

For men who have been subjected to sexual abuse, and who also experience same-sex desire, this can add to self-blame. This can invite men to attribute any same-sex feeling, confusion, desire or action to the sexual abuse (O'Leary 1999, p. 52).

> I thought it was something about me, that I must deserve this. I worried that I might be gay. I thought, that because men have done this stuff to me, does this make me gay? Like my identity was decided for me.

Finding a way through the silencing and intimidating tactics of homophobia is complex. Often for men to be aware of other men's experience can help to alleviate some of the isolation and shame that homophobia can cultivate. Sometimes the physiological stimulation that some men may experience at the time of the abuse can create confusion and shame. Professionals can offer information about the fact that many males may experience an erection or ejaculation while the abuse is occurring. These physiological reactions are responses to physical contact, and are not indicative in any way of consent (Lew 1990). This information can facilitate a conversation that differentiates between physiological responses and the man's emotional response to the abuse. Additionally it is important that professionals find ways to challenge the destructive influence of homophobia.

Further conversations can help the man to focus on the perpetrator's misuse of power, rather than the actual sexual acts involved in the abuse. Within this it is important to note that the sexuality of men who sexually abuse is not the issue, their identity is separate and overshadowed by their acts of abuse. In this way it can be acknowledged that sexual identity is not pre-determined by someone else's violent and abusive acts. For many men regardless of whether or not they have been sexually abused, it can be complex to work through whether or not they are straight, gay or bisexual. In this way it is important to open up space for men to take the opportunity to talk about sexuality (straight, gay or bisexual) as legitimate choices in the realm of delight, love, hope and pride.

Stories of resilience and hope

For many men the community portrayal and ongoing effects of childhood sexual abuse can erode their hope.

> The media image of guys who have been abused is often that his whole life is wrecked. This doesn't give us hope. Because basically, we need inspirational work and stories to be told, because otherwise we get the sense that we can't deal with things, that we don't have it within ourselves. It's sort of like a constant underestimation of our ability to deal with things, and to find peace in the midst of it all, in the midst of the pain and suffering.

It can be important for men to re-tell aspects of their experiences that may have been obscured by the perpetrator's use of power and manipulation, as well as the effects of self-blame and confusion. As conversations develop recollections about experiences of abuse can be re-told with knowledge about the dynamics of power. The following is an example of a man's recollection of feeling inadequate about resisting the abuse; this conversation offered an opportunity for hope in the re-telling of the story:

> Whenever he'd take me to the bathroom I would fight him and struggle with him to get away from him, but I was a little kid, and he was a big 20 year old, yeah, he was very strong. And I never won those battles . . . I have never been able to beat him.

Recollections such as this can give the practitioner an opportunity to question the man more about how the re-telling of the story may have changed. Conversations may highlight the imbalance in power, and the courage it took to stand against such odds.

> I was a shit of a kid, like an outcast. I hoped that Mum would realise what was happening. But I couldn't say anything. My stepdad said if I told he'd kill me. I cried all night.

Quite often men's acts of resilience have been hidden or negatively internalised. Sometimes in the re-telling of the experience acts of resistance, protest and connection offer opportunities for hope to emerge (O'Leary 1998). Helping men to uncover past and present acts that have led to their survival can be liberating. The above quote provides an example of an opportunity where such acts can be positively reclaimed. For example, past behaviour that may have been internalised as delinquency, can be understood in the context of resistance. Past thoughts of hope for help can stimulate conversations about resilience and connection. Simple acts like crying during the abuse may have been internalised as 'weak', where in actual fact crying is an overt sign of protest about what is happening. These recollections of coping with effects of abuse in the past and present can help to clarify future desires.

Advice to professionals

> The main thing that helped was talking about it and knowing that I was believed. He gave me hope that I can overcome the cards that have been dealt to me, and become something I want to become.

In my research, men were keen to offer advice to professionals. For some of them their initial experience with professionals had not been helpful. Sometimes psychopathology became the focus of the professional, rather than hearing the man's experience and the significance of the struggle he was presenting. Some men spoke about their involvement in psychiatric services that did not allow adequate space for their experience to be understood. In some cases the men's fears about disclosure were realised in the professional's response.

Men expected that professionals be aware of the many issues that they may face and that professionals create a non–judgmental environment, but also a context where the professional did not detach themselves from their own feelings. One man offered this advice to professionals:

> Don't be judgmental. It's a long hard row, I know, but it's worth-while. But the trouble with some professionals is they sit back like cold ivory towers and detach their feelings, and that's wrong.

Men suggested that professionals need to show faith in them, even during times when men may appear to be lost, confused or feeling hopeless. For men to know that they can trust a professional who will gently persist with them can be enormously encouraging. One man best summed this up:

> Professionals need to know that we are afraid and vulnerable. They need patience, that if we miss appointments, that if we seem to go backwards, that if we seem to go over and over the same

ground, that if we feel hopeless, we need not to be rejected, we need to be accepted. And for better or worse, you, the counsellor is the person, you know and you need to stay with us, because we are talking about it. So do things that can affirm and build on trust. It doesn't mean you don't challenge us. Because I have appreciated those challenges, even though they are hard. It is a scary thing to do, to speak about this stuff. It's unknown territory.

Some broader implications for addressing male sexual victimisation

Human service organisations can also respond to male sexual victimisation by raising community awareness. Many men in my research interviews commented on the need for public recognition of male sexual victimisation. Ensuring that publicity is accurate and sensitive to men's experiences is important. One man explained how greater societal awareness of sexual abuse of males would have made a difference to his experience:

> If it was more public I would have spoken about it a lot earlier. If it was more public in a structural sense, that sexual abuse does happen to males, and if we created opportunities for men to talk about it, it'd be harder for the men that do it to get away with it.

Human service professionals can challenge issues such as homophobia, which can be a major restraint to disclosure. One man, who thought that a world free from homophobia would make a difference to the occurrence of sexual abuse, identified the power of homophobia:

> I'll tell you right now, if we get rid of homophobia, sexual abuse would come right down. Because it's the heterosexual population that abuse children, mostly, I'm not saying homosexuals don't. But, if we didn't have homophobia you wouldn't be able to intimidate small boys, pre-pubescent boys wouldn't be intimidated, and teenagers would not be intimidated. You wouldn't have teenage boys intimidating other teenage boys by calling them poofters and being too scared to talk.

Programs that challenge homophobia can also have an important influence on the ease at which males can name sexual abuse. Trudinger *et al.* (1998) have developed workshops for young men that deconstruct some of the myths of homophobia and masculinity. Initiatives such as this can help to create safer environments for males to discuss issues such as sexual abuse.

Fostering community awareness of male sexual victimisation requires ongoing strategies that cater for the many diverse groups of men. These groups in Australia would include men from a non-heterosexual orientation, Indigenous Australian men, men from migrant or ethnic minorities and men living with psychiatric diagnosis or disabilities. Some community organisations have successfully produced information leaflets, books and posters, while organisations that specialise in working with males who have experienced childhood sexual abuse can offer training opportunities to other human service professionals.

CONCLUSION

Human service professionals who work with men in many diverse fields of practice need to recognise that a significant proportion of their client group may have been sexually abused. Being aware of the potential difficulties these men may face is important in offering services that create opportunities for men to speak about their experiences. The scrutiny and many of the difficulties that men experience are embedded in our dominant cultural practices that extend privileges to certain stereotyped masculinities. As more and more men speak out about sexual abuse, the experience of victims will gain greater acceptance and respect; it is with this awareness that the actions of those men who use sexual violence against others will be justifiably placed under more intense scrutiny. Community awareness about male victims of childhood sexual abuse needs to come primarily from us as men. While male sexual violence continues to be perpetrated against males, it diminishes the hope that male violence will cease against women and children. It is perhaps not only men's responsibility to themselves, but also their responsibility to women and children that men speak about sexual violence.

Human service professionals have some prime opportunities to uncloak male sexual victimisation from the tyranny of myths and silence. This chapter has attempted to introduce human service professionals to the many complexities that males may face when dealing with an experience of childhood sexual abuse. The ideas presented form a foundation from which practitioners can respond to men sensitively and empathically.

8 | Men and mental health: Counselling men with a psychiatric disability

Peter Humphries

In this chapter I will reflect on my experience in counselling men, particularly in a mental health context. It is, of course, impossible to generalise about a group as large and diverse as men. As Pease (1999c, p. 99) observes 'we cannot speak of masculinity as a singular term, but rather should explore masculinities'. In talking about men there are differences in age, class, culture, sexuality and race that all introduce an infinite range of variables. It is the process by which men 'position' themselves in this multiplicity of discourses and how they can be influenced by counselling that I want to explore.

PSYCHIATRIC DIAGNOSIS AND MENTAL HEALTH

Much of the work I have done with men has been while I have been working in mental health services and I would like to consider some issues that arise from this context before moving on to look at the process of counselling men.

There have been some undeniable advances in the delivery of mental health services in Australia and other parts of the world over the past 30 years. The main improvement has been in the gradual closure of the many large psychiatric hospitals and a move to the delivery of mental health services in the community. The arguments for the delivery of services to people where they actually live are for me almost irrefutable (although this perspective is not without its critics). However, my own view is that progress has not been as great as we would like to believe, as the same models of mental health care seem to have survived the shift to the community pretty much intact. The view is still prevalent that people with a psychiatric disability are suffering from an 'illness' that needs to be 'diagnosed' and 'treated' with little regard to the actual needs and circumstances of the individual. Foucault (1967) saw the development of psychiatry as an exercise in power and that this power creates its own 'reality'. The use of such terms as 'assertive follow up' to describe the treatment of an individual without their consent is evidence of this. This is not to say that there are occasions where a person does need some treatment and protection as a result of an active psychosis. It is the manner, however, in which this coercive treatment approach has been accepted in many services without any awareness of what is actually happening, that is, the use of a form of institutional power over an individual, which is the concern.

One of the big challenges for me in working with clients in a mental health context has been the struggle in assisting them to not see their life situation as defined by their diagnosis and waiting for the expert to find the appropriate treatment that will 'cure' them. This belief in this definition of their life leads many to become passive in their pursuit of alternative ways of being. Men have been more likely than women to just accept this external view of their situation and as a result allow themselves to do nothing to change what is happening to them. My explanation for this is that women often maintain their personal networks more effectively in a time of crisis, while men are more likely to attempt to sort the problem out alone as part of their view of 'competence'. For me then, the first challenge in working with a man has been to assist him to see the possibilities that remain for him and not to define himself as being his 'diagnosis'. This is a reflection on the continuing power of psychiatry to dominate the delivery of mental health services. I would not like to overstate this as there are many compassionate and innovative psychiatrists and nurses who are also doing what they can to overcome this dominant ideology. There can be no doubt, when looking at our mental health services, that the power of this solely biological view of psychiatric disability remains intact. The point is often made that the use of diagnostic categories helps us make some sense of complex and difficult situations and while this can be true to a point, it is difficult, in my experience, for many mental health professionals to resist this dynamic of generalising everything about the individual from the diagnostic label applied to them.

PSYCHIATRIC DIAGNOSIS AND GENDER

A recent Australian study of the incidence and severity of 'psychotic illness' (Jablensky *et al.* 1999) indicates that men are more likely than women to be diagnosed as having a psychotic disorder and to experience more severe symptoms for a longer period of time. Generally, the explanations regarding this are couched in the same biological terms as is much of the research concerned with isolating the 'causes' of these disorders. My own sense is that the social construction of gender is a factor in this as well and has something to do with the observation I made earlier regarding men being more likely than women to define themselves in terms of a psychiatric diagnosis once it is given. I suspect that the extreme passivity so often evident in young men who have been diagnosed with a 'psychotic illness' is as much a product of the failure they feel as men who are no longer in 'control' as it is of the symptomotology that may result from their 'illness'. This line of thinking raises many interesting questions that need further thought and research.

Jimenez (1997) reviews the psychiatric conceptions of mental disorders in women and concludes that the psychiatric diagnoses introduced in the last 30 years indicate that a psychological model has replaced the biological model through which psychiatry views women's experience. In particular, she observes that the introduction of the diagnosis 'borderline personality disorder' with its cluster of 'feminine characteristics' in its criteria, is indicative of how mainstream psychiatry stereotypes and limits the experience of women in our society and reasserts dominant values. There are estimates that three-quarters of the people who receive this diagnosis are women (Widigier & Weissman 1991) and suggestions as to the gender bias inherent in the process of psychiatric diagnosis are beginning to emerge (Spock *et al.* 1990).

ANTI-OPPRESSIVE PRACTICE

The literature on counselling men has only begun to appear over the past couple of decades. We have seen an increasing awareness among men working in this field of how traditional counselling approaches, that lack any real gender awareness or analysis, run the risk of reinforcing oppressive and often violent behaviour on the part of men. In particular, this can happen as the counsellor unwittingly colludes with the man to 'explain' away his violent behaviour. It is very important to place the counselling of men in a framework that explicitly rejects violence and is built on a foundation of assisting men to develop a masculinity based on cooperation and equality and not domination and fear.

This anti-oppressive or pro-feminist approach to working with men has not been overtly included as yet within mainstream counselling approaches. Pringle (1995), in considering the development of family therapy over the last 30 years, observes some key themes evident in many other developing areas of counselling practice as well. He sees that family therapy has developed a marked technical ethos, is dominated by men, and has created for them valuable 'career passports'. For Pringle, any therapy that does not incorporate the dimension of power, becomes a part of the problem and not the solution. Pease (1997, p. 98) is rightly concerned that unless the approach to working with men is 'guided by the primary goal of ending violence against women then they may reinforce the controlling and coercive behaviours and attitudes of men who are violent'. It is very important that the approach to counselling men I outline below is recognised as being built on the understanding that men need to be responsible for their actions and behaviour. One of the key benefits of the counselling process is that it provides the opportunity for men to become aware of the impact of violent and oppressive practices on others and to recognise that violence works for no one. Wolf-Light (1999) shares my optimism for the effectiveness of anti-oppressive counselling practice. His approach is built on four basic principles: responsibility, vulnerability, empathy and creativity. The development of these qualities is essential to enable the development of a non-oppressive masculinity, and it is even more important for men who are feeling defeated and angry as a result of their experience of a psychiatric disability.

COUNSELLING AND PSYCHOTHERAPY

The process of assisting a man to see the possibilities that exist for him beyond his 'diagnosis' involves the engagement of the man in counselling or psychotherapy. I do not think it would be useful for my purposes here to get into a lengthy debate concerning the difference between counselling and psychotherapy. In essence I agree with Rowan (1997) that there is very little to differentiate the two and I will use the terms interchangeably. I am attracted, however, to the meaning of psychotherapy when taken from its two Greek roots, that is, the healing of the soul. For much of the past 50 years the whole field of counselling and psychotherapy has been dominated by a struggle for supremacy by the various schools of thought. We have seen this manifested in the vast literature that has been generated in the name of 'research' that purports to prove the efficacy of one approach over the others. In fact the only variable that is consistent in all this research is that the quality of the relationship that is developed between the worker and the client is the essential determinant of a successful 'outcome' (Orlinsky et al. 1994; Mazioli & Alexander 1991). Of course, the whole notion of an outcome in a process that involves so many variables is to oversimplify the whole thing to almost the point of meaninglessness. My experience has been that counselling and psychotherapy are essential in any effort to assist a man to move beyond seeing himself in pathological terms. One of the main difficulties with the wholehearted acceptance by a man of a psychiatric diagnosis is that it counteracts any efforts the man may make to accept some responsibility for his life and circumstances.

Psychotherapy of course has its detractors, and certainly it is a process that can be used to exploit others or simply be done badly. Eysenck's attack on psychotherapy in 1952 is still the best known. In this paper Eysenck attempted to show that two-thirds of patients treated with various forms of psychotherapy got better as did two-thirds of patients who were merely placed on a waiting list. This, in Eysenck's view, demonstrated that psychotherapy did not work and was in fact an expensive waste of time. This study has been often refuted (as Rowan 1997 observes) and while there is little 'evidence' that one approach to counselling and psychother-apy is better than another there is 'evidence' that the process itself can make a difference (see, for example, Barkham 1992).

A common criticism of psychotherapy is that it tends to work only with the 'worried well', that is, those people who are already socially integrated and probably would survive reasonably well with or without psychotherapy. Many mainstream texts on abnormal psychology see any form of counselling or psychotherapy as con-traindicated when any form of psychiatric problem is present, in the belief that the individual in this situation is so affected that the process is at best a waste of time and at worst harmful. This has certainly not been my experience. Over time, I have become completely convinced that there is no substitute for a trusting and supportive ongoing relationship between a worker and client in ensuring a positive outcome for a person with a psychiatric disability. It is to this process, particularly in the context of working with men who have attracted a psychiatric diagnosis, that I now want to turn.

THE COUNSELLING PROCESS

A lot has been written about how men do not like or trust counselling as a process. Donovan Research (1999) in a report for the Australian Attorney General's Department on counselling men stated that men generally see counselling as not working and that it is seen as the 'last resort'. They go on to make the point that men see themselves as competent and self-reliant in the world and as a result are not in need of assistance, regardless of the situation. My experience leads me to agree with both these points, as I have found men to initially be very suspicious of counselling and to be reluctant to concede that they are not coping in any way. The key word here of course is 'initially'. The manner in which the man is engaged in the counselling process, and the expectations of it that he develops, are of vital importance. For me, one of the enduring myths in counselling men is that, by their nature, men respond favourably to brief, direct, solution-focused approaches. We are told that men want to get in there and out again the moment the crisis has passed. This is not surprising, given, as we have noted, that men do not have a positive view of counselling, and that the nature of the process is contrary to the need to feel in control of your life. My concern with then offering a man a short, sharp, solution-focused approach is that the counsellor is then colluding with the man to reinforce this view of masculinity. This does not mean there won't be times where this approach is appropriate; however, generally speaking, when a man arrives at a mental health service, usually as the result of some major crisis, he is already past the point of being able to benefit from a 'quick fix'. In this context I am in complete agreement with Rowan (1997, p. 108) when he observes that 'the longer the problem has been in existence, the longer it will take to deal with'.

GETTING STARTED AND BUILDING TRUST

Whenever I have been asked to explain the process of counselling I have tended to borrow heavily on the stages that Chaplin (1988) utilises. Chaplin offers a clear overview of how a counselling relationship should develop, based on feminist values, that is, not advocating a particular technique or approach as being the 'method' that will lead to success. In my view, counselling and psychotherapy have suffered greatly at the hands of those self-appointed 'experts' who present, with certainty, that their technique or approach will succeed in all situations. Counselling is not just a matter of technique; it is an interaction between two human beings that is built on trust and mutual respect. Chaplin's work later formed the basis for Rowan's (1997) work in which counselling is seen as an 'initiation' process in which men can mature and grow. While mystical at times in tone, Rowan's work is also informed by a strong profeminist perspective.

Trust is developed in counselling in the same manner it is developed anywhere else. You trust someone when you feel that they are being honest with you, not judging you and open to hearing and understanding your point of view. It is always important to be clear about the boundaries that surround the relationship and that both parties are clear on what they expect of the other. I have consistently found that men respond positively to an open and honest exchange of views and that doing this facilitates the building of trust. This is particularly important in situations where other people have been harmed or are potentially at risk. Without the worker being clear from the beginning that any form of violent or intimidating behaviour is unacceptable there is always the risk of colluding with the man not accepting responsibility for his behaviour. This appears to be a very straightforward concept but I have found it can become very difficult when the man, his family and often other workers are busy explaining away violent behaviour in terms of the man's diagnosis, particularly when some form of psychosis is involved.

Engaging with a man who is suspicious and may even be hostile to you takes time and beginning with some exploration of why the man feels this way is generally a good start. Often you will find some fear of talking to someone unknown and an embarrassment about being in the situation in the first place, given that men should always be in control. I have found it very useful to acknowledge that men often do find these situations more difficult to deal with than women and that the man's job is to question me, and get to know me, to the point where he can feel confident in working with me. I often make it plain that this may take a little time and hope he does not initially judge me too harshly. I also explore what has worked in dealing with these issues in the past and generally get the answer that nothing, or little 'has worked'. I then offer the assurance that as far as I can I will keep working with the man for as long as he feels the need. I have often been surprised at the power this simple statement of commitment can have.

IDENTIFYING THEMES

Identifying themes is simply allowing the man to tell you what is going on for him and how he sees it may all be connected. Are there any patterns he has noticed and what is he wanting to be different? The identifying of themes can occur quite quickly at times but generally speaking this will take at least a couple of sessions and you will need to assist in the development of a framework that enables the man to see his experience as a whole. This means it is very important for the worker to resist the temptation to seize on an issue and define it as 'the problem'. This is a critical point. So often there is pressure for the worker to quickly decide what the issue is and, often more importantly, if it is then appropriate for that particular agency. There is a strong dynamic at work to divide up experience into neat little packages rather than taking the time to sec the whole. The damage that this can do early in a counselling process is obvious and generally further convinces the man that he will not be heard here.

Identifying themes is about allowing the man to genuinely review where he is in his life and again, my experience has been that to focus too quickly on one particular issue or area removes the vitality from what is happening. How often do we learn in counselling work that things are often not what they seem at first? One of the difficulties in a mental health context, is, of course, that the problem has often been already defined by the 'diagnosis' and it can take some time to encourage a man to see beyond the label that has been assigned to him. You can be met with a situation where the man will tell you that his family life is disintegrating, he has lost his job and he feels frightened in any social situation but what he wants you to tell him is how he can 'fix' the 'chemical imbalance' that is causing his 'depression'.

EXPLORING THE PAST

Exploring the past gives the man the opportunity to look at his life up to now and to make what connections he can between where he is now and what has happened to him in the past. I tend to particularly encourage the man to tell me about the family he grew up in and ask him to reflect on what part of who he is now grew from that time. It can also be important to allow the man to tell you a little about the significant relationships he has had as an adult. Quite often I have met men who can happily tell you how they have entered into a relationship with another woman every two years or so and see this as them just not meeting the right person, rather than asking what it is about them and the way they view women that makes sustaining a relationship so difficult. The challenge in exploring the past is to do it in such a way that the man can see the possibilities for growth and change in his life rather than believing that his future is already pre-determined by his past. In essence, the past does matter and this is one reason why I can be a bit suspicious of approaches that merely emphasise the 'here and now'. Part of taking responsibility for our lives is acknowledging and accepting our past and the part we have played in what has occurred.

FACING AMBIVALENCE

Chaplin (1988) calls the next stage of the counselling process facing ambivalence. Essentially this is about all of us accepting the opposites that make up our personalities, for example the happy and the sad, the kind and the cruel. As themes are identified and the links with our past acknowledged we are faced with what to do with all of this. My experience has been that many men do find the whole process of self-acceptance difficult as they often have an 'ideal type' in mind of what sort of man they should be and accepting that they have fallen short of this is very hard to do. They can often at this time become disenchanted with the counselling process and become very critical of the worker. It is crucial that the worker is able to accept the criticism being made of him or her as an important part of the process. No longer seeing the worker as the perfect person who is the answer to his problems is the beginning of the man accepting his own faults and flaws. Self-acceptance is the platform for real change and I do not think any sustainable change can occur without it. With a man whose sense of self has been badly damaged as he has internalised a view of himself as say 'schizophrenic' the time needs to be spent enabling the man to reclaim other positive parts of himself. I have often found encouraging a man to again take up something he was once good at can be of help here.

MAKING CHANGES

Once a man has been given the opportunity to explore what is happening in his life, what influence the past has on his life and has begun to accept who he is, you have the foundation for genuine change. For me this is where many of the cognitive techniques that focus on problem-solving actually fit. Your hope is that you are now working with a man who is in a position to make decisions about what he wants to change in his life and how he is going to do it. The difference in the process I have just briefly outlined, and more short-term targeted interventions, is that in this process we have taken the time to assist the man to accept that he can take responsibility and make his life better. To move to this position prematurely is to display a lack of care that ultimately undermines the process itself.

IMPLICATIONS FOR SERVICE DELIVERY

The argument will undoubtedly be raised that this is all very well but in my mental health service there just is no time to work in this manner. I readily acknowledge the pressures so many public mental health services face with diminishing resources and increased demand to provide an effective service. I can only hope that the argument for effective service delivery can assist in these situations in the recognition that even the briefest of interventions is a waste of money if it is of no benefit to the client. Men with a psychiatric disability are no different to any other men in that we all desper-ately need intimacy and connectedness with others. As men, we are so often not given the tools we need to relate to others. My commitment to the psychotherapeutic approach I have outlined comes from my experience that it is only through this level of contact that we can genuinely assist a man experiencing a psychiatric disability to reconstruct his life. For me this is at least worth striving for, particularly when faced with the deterministic and pathologised approach that can represent the accepted approach to community mental health practice in so many places.

CONCLUSION

In this chapter I have outlined an approach to working with men in a mental health context that relies heavily on developing a trusting and honest therapeutic relationship over time. The essential challenge is to assist the man to not define himself in terms of the psychiatric diagnosis he has attracted and this can only be done by the worker 'journeying' with the man as he develops a broader, more positive and open view of his world. This can at times be challenging as together you face the fear and anxiety that can come from letting go of old and established ways of being. In the safety of a therapeutic setting a man can learn that he can develop intimacy with another human being without losing his own identity. He can take the opportunity to reflect on the values and beliefs that have governed his life up to now and move to a more open and non-oppressive view of how men and women relate to each other. For me, working in this way is a powerful response to the at times still prevalent belief that the person is indistinguishable from their symptomatology. This is particularly important in working with men as we strive for genuine autonomy, intimacy and connectedness with others.

PART III

GENDER-BASED APPROACHES TO WORKING WITH MALE OFFENDERS

9 | Men and child protection: Developing new kinds of relationships between men and children

Mary Hood

Child protection is an issue that developed societies currently focus much attention, concern and resources on. There is a community consensus that we do not want to have children exposed to neglect or harsh physical or emotional abuse, nor have pre-pubertal children involved in sexual activity. This level of attention to child protection is relatively new, not because we love our children more, but because of different ways of thinking about women and children and their treatment within our societies.

Child abuse was created as an issue of community concern in the 1970s and 1980s, largely emanating from the work of feminists challenging the subordinate place of women in society and in the family. As part of this, the women's movement brought into public gaze the most extreme forms of male domination—physical and sexual violence towards women and children within the formerly private confines of the home. Once exposed, the majority of our community acknowledged that men did not have the right to control women and to abuse women and children emotionally, physically and sexually. Government policies, laws and programs were developed to confront abusive men, both legally and thera-peutically.

Efforts to investigate, ameliorate and prevent further child abuse (and sexual abuse in particular) were initially developed from the feminist theoretical framework. This strongly portrayed child abuse as a male versus female issue, caused by men and resulting from the patriarchal structures of the society they controlled. Not all agreed with this position, however. Medical specialists, who had been instrumental in drawing public attention to physical injury in infants, promoted a more psychiatric non-gendered perspective on the causes and therefore the remedies. The legal 'paternity' also found much to oppose in the feminist construction of the issues when asked to implement charges of child sexual and physical assault against men in courts of law.

There is considerable evidence to support the feminist position. While women do commit neglect of children, feminism can argue with justification that the modern patriarchal society fails to provide adequate social and financial resources to enable stressed, isolated women to raise their children. Even if we accept lavish estimates that allocate physical and emotional child abuse to men and women at around 50 per cent, men spend so little time with children compared to women as to put these figures in bold perspective. As well, the empirical research identifies males overwhelmingly as the source of sexual abuse of children (Finkelhor *et al.* 1990), and also of the more violent incidents of physical abuse. Violence to mothers is also seen as linked to multiple types of abuse of the children within the family (Stanley & Goddard 1993).

Acknowledgment of the feminist construction of men as responsible for child abuse has had some consequences for the relationships of non-abusing men with children and society as a whole. A side effect has been to cast a shadow over the interaction of all men with all children. Community and child protection policies and practices of the past decade have responded strongly to the implications of men's role in child abuse. Child-care centres and schools have designed programs to ensure that lone men are supervised in the company of children and adolescents at all times. Child welfare foster care and mentoring programs rarely allow men to provide primary care for children and even advise them not to be alone in the house with an unrelated child. In child protection investigations, all the men in the environment of an allegedly abused child tend to come under suspicion. Sometimes a troubled child has unjustly accused a male of sexual behaviour, and once an allegation has been made, it is very difficult to prove that abuse did not occur, so that a stigma remains with the innocent as well as the guilty. As a result, many men feel they are under suspicion by just approaching a child, and that they are prevented from full, nurturing, reciprocal relationships with children by the current social attitude. This has created real dilemmas for men in child protection work, for men in families and for men in all their relationships with children.

There is a paradox here for feminist aims as well. Some sections of the women's movement wanted men to assume a fair share of the responsibility for child-rearing, so women could more fully participate in the world outside the home. While many men have been willing to become more involved with their own and other people's children, they do so under this increased shadow of mistrust. Community group leaders, male teachers and sports coaches are some of the men affected. Custodial and non-custodial fathers trying to maintain contact with their children after divorce also feel this dilemma strongly. It is important that in raising the awareness about untrustworthy men who do abuse children, resulting policies and practices do not further alienate all men from understanding children and their needs.

The data on male child abusers are recognised as incomplete and it may never be possible to get accurate information because of difficulties defining abuse and substantiating allegations. The lack of precise knowledge contributes to the generalised anxiety by allowing exaggeration of the dangers. However, Pringle (1995, p. 170) concludes after reviewing the evidence that 'a very significant minority of the male population sexually assaults girls and boys as well as women'. On the one hand there is a need to think realistically about the percentage of men who actually do physical or sexual harm to children and to find out whether the abuse is intentional or accidental or through ignorance. This allows useful responses to specific situations. On the other hand, the construction of masculinity that allows 'a significant minority' of men to abuse children in this way needs to be challenged.

So it is important not just to throw more men, unprepared, into relationships with young children and hope abuse does not occur. If men are to become more involved in interactions with young children, they need to understand the effects of abusive and oppressive behaviour on children, but also the attitudes that allow the abusive behaviour to occur. In this chapter it is intended to look more closely at these two aspects of men's interactions with children and to suggest if and how it is possible to develop new kinds of relationships between them. Also considered is how men who work in child protection areas can contribute to this process personally and in their work.

THE EFFECT OF ABUSIVE BEHAVIOUR ON CHILDREN

Examining the effects of men's abusive behaviour towards children and adolescents might give some clues about what needs to change. Most current discussions of child abuse use four headings: neglect, physical abuse, sexual abuse and emotional abuse. The physical signs of burns, beatings, sexual assault and chronic neglect are obvious. But the more we learn from children and adult survivors of all the kinds of abuse, the more we realise that emotional and developmental repercussions often outweigh any physical impact at the time.

- Blame and denigration of the child may cause guilt, shame, lowered self-esteem and a sense of difference from others, leading to isolation, drug or alcohol abuse, selfmutilation or suicide.
- Betrayal of trust may cause grief, depression, extreme dependency and anger. The child may also not learn the ability to judge trustworthiness in others, yet show discomfort or aggression as relationships become closer.
- Powerlessness in the abuse situation may cause anxiety, fear, a sense of inefficacy in the child. This can be expressed behaviourally as identification with the abuser, depression and even dissociation.
- Premature sexualisation may cause the child confusion about sexual identity and norms, inability to separate sex from affection or disgust of any sex or intimacy. Precocious sexual activity, preoccupation with sex, prostitution, or avoidance of intimate relationships and the experiencing of flashback memories can result (adapted from Finkelhor 1984.).

Of course, some emotional effects may lead to very physical consequences, including the development of somatic complaints and phobias in children and adolescents. Researchers (Perry *et al.* 1995) also believe that during the first year of life, the baby experiences behavioural and emotional 'states' in response to parental nurturing, which are then laid down in the brain as permanent 'traits', influencing future intellectual and behavioural capabilities. Chronically violent or unreliable responses by a parent result in less than optimal coping and learning abilities in the baby.

Therefore, current child protection therapeutic work holds that, while the physical effects of neglect, direct physical violence and sexual assault on children are obviously serious and must be prevented or mended, the emotional effects of these negative behaviours towards children are crucial and must not be ignored. Emotional effects tend to be long-lasting and life-defining and not only prevent the individual child from reaching their full potential, but influence second and third generations of children in cycles of abusive behaviour, if not understood and resolved. This latter process of resolution (abused children gaining the confidence and self-esteem to believe they should not have been treated in that way) is crucial to them being able to decide to act differently from their abusers as they grow into adults (Egeland, Jacobvitz & Sroufe 1988).

Many abused children have overcome the extra burden imposed on them by such difficult emotions and achieved successful lives in all areas. However, too many others have continued to struggle with issues of self-esteem, emotional attachment, lack of ability to trust others, and been prevented from finding personal fulfilment in their adult lives. A few have acted out the abuse they suffered on others.

WHAT ATTITUDES CONTRIBUTE TO MEN ABUSING CHILDREN?

People who abuse children seem not to have developed (or suspend) the ability to put themselves in the child's place and feel the hurt, the fear, the sorrow and the confusion the child feels during and following abuse. The abuser acts very much from egocentric impulses and emotions.

For the last half-century in Western societies men have been progressively separated from child-rearing roles. After the Second World War, a clear division of roles between men and women was reinforced in an attempt to provide stability and ease men back into a 'normal' society. Women were allocated the practical day-to-day child-rearing responsibilities, men given the responsibility and power of being the head of the family in return for providing its financial support. Early American sociologists such as Parsons and Bales (1955) were influential in legitimising these differing mother and father roles, and Bowlby's (1958) work on infant attachment stressed the importance of mothers to the healthy emotional and psychological development of the infant. As economic development was given primary importance, many faced longer working hours. Work weary men were not to be 'bothered' with the 'minor' issues of the family and developed a culture of relaxation away from the family home. Increased mobility weakened the influence of male extended family and community supports. Children were not needed in the workforce and remained in school longer, increasing their separation from their fathers and male work environments.

However, these constructions of male–female roles and the male head of family life did not stay relevant for long. Children were subject to social influences wider than their parents through their education, through the development of medical and psychological professional opinion and through the mass media, which introduced popular and marketable trends and ideas. All these forces challenged the influence and authority of the male head of the family. From the 1970s on, when the women's movement emerged, changes such as work for women outside the home, alternative support to women and their children through government benefits, women's control of reproduction, all continued to challenge the construction of men's role in the family.

Along with this movement reducing the authority of men's role within the family, the image of masculinity has become more exaggerated and unrealistic, strongly reinforced by the pervasive modern media. An essential part of the current construction of heterosexual masculinity is the rejection of the feminine, specifically the attributes of nurturing, emotional openness, intimacy and a willingness to be dependent (Pringle 1995). In one analysis, Smith (1996) identifies eight dichotomies that distinguish the construction of masculinity: masculinity vs femininity; rational vs emotional; universal vs particular; mind vs body; higher vs lower; separate vs connected; individual vs collective; inadequacy vs development. The 'ideal' man is untouched by emotions, holding to universal principles, competing with others, ignoring bodily pain and pleasure, resilient, independent and all this believed to be innate to the 'true' male. With ideas of manhood described negatively rather than positively, a constant threat of 'insufficiency' exists for men, pushing them to deny emotions, to disregard the personal experience of others, to be 'in control' and not need to listen or ask for help. Men unaware of their body and their emotions are more likely to attribute any feelings that arise in them to other people, to feel justified in personalising and then reacting to the impact of those feelings on them (Smith 1996, p. 42).

The social forces mentioned have made it more difficult for individual men to learn empathy for children as they spend less time engaged in children's concerns and are emotionally estranged from them. Those men confused about their own masculinity and expectations of them as fathers can become more focused on their own hurts, needs and wants than on those of a child. Abusive men have not understood their own feelings and their causes so as to control them nor, as Jenkins (1990) sees it, to take personal responsibility for their actions. For example, a man, insecure in his masculinity, whose wife leaves and divorces him, may feel wronged and humiliated as well as justified in abusing their children to make her feel sorry. Or, a young isolated male adolescent, whose sexuality is just developing, may become obsessive about the pornographic videos he has obtained and abuse the eight-year-old girl from next door, with no thought for her experience.

A lack of knowledge about infant and child development also contributes to some abusive incidents. Many of the deaths and injuries of young babies have been inflicted by young men who cannot stand the stress of an infant's demanding cry. In a common scenario the exhausted new mother makes demands on the new father (who never planned to have a child) to care for the two-month-old baby for a few hours, so she can rest. He feels inadequate in this new relationship and responsibility. When the baby responds to his tension, lack of knowledge and sensitivity by crying, the new father is unable to think of the infant and unaware of its physical vulnerability. He shakes the baby until it stops, causing brain damage or death. Knowledge about babies is not innate.

DO CHILDREN NEED RELATIONSHIPS WITH MEN?

Do families need fathers? Many assert this to be so, although it seems on ideology rather than evidence. Female lone parents have difficulties without male partners in terms of low income, poor housing and lack of child-care support. But while there are links between poverty, crime and unemployment and the absence of fathers in poor families, these are correlations not causal relationships.

Do children need a parent of the same gender? Pringle concludes his review of this question saying 'there is evidence that children of both genders fare just as well emotionally and developmentally in families without men' (1995). He quotes a study of children raised by lone fathers and mothers that concluded (Phillips 1993, in Pringle 1995 p. 73):

> . . . while it is clearly an advantage for a growing child to have a
> close relationship with an adult of the same gender, that is not as
> important in the long run as a relationship with a parent who loves
> them and isn't afraid to show it.

Masculine role models within the family will only be useful if they are showing children the attitudes and behaviour that it is hoped they will learn. If we aspire to create a more positive, less violent and sexually equal society, children in contact with men who model nurturing, empathic behaviour will assist with this. The most enduring change in social behaviour between men, women and children comes not just from changing laws or from adult education, but from inculcating the new generation of children with the experience of behaviour by both sexes. Boys can use contact with males who model sensitive and nurturing behaviour to grow to be men who do the same. Girls can use such early relationships with men to develop strong and clear expectations of reciprocal and equal relationships with men in their adult lives.

RAISING BOYS DIFFERENTLY

Many have noted that our society's current approach to raising boys contributes to their difficulties in social behaviour and relationships in adolescent and adult life. Kindlon and Thompson (1999) talk of a key concept, the 'emotional illiteracy' of boys, a lack of a vocabulary with which to talk about feelings. This occurs through adults reinforcing, in subtle but very influential ways, the mental construction of masculinity in which boys should not display emotions. For example, mothers and fathers tend to discuss with their daughter the feelings that might lie behind another child crying but would be more likely to ignore or only briefly acknowledge it with their son. Most adults do tend to give less comforting attention to a boy who is crying than to a girl. We expect boys to overcome their fears, but allow girls to avoid them. Emotionally constrained fathers model emotional distance to sons, and even shame boys who show 'weakness' through emotional expression. When such signals are primary, boys learn to deny emotion or turn it into anger, leading to the poorer ability to predict, prevent and respond to difficult emotional situations. Emotionally literate boys need modelling, teaching and discussion from all.

As mentioned earlier, an essential part of the current construction of heterosexual masculinity is the rejection of the feminine. Such myths of masculinity have led to the premature separation of boys from their mothers and from emotional support in general (Silverstein & Rashbaum 1994). Alongside fear of the 'feminine' traits is a belief that disconnection is important in order to become independent and 'a man'. Pollack says (1998, p. xxiv):

> As early as five or six many boys are pushed out of the family and expected to become independent—in . . . situations they may not be ready to handle. We give our boys in early adolescence a second shove—into new schools, sports competitions, jobs, dating, travel and more.

This early separation from mothers can lead to a feeling of abandonment or 'unrequited love' and hasten the emotional shutting down process, as well as distract from other development. Most boys do not have fathers who fill this void. Boys need an end to this premature separation from intimacy and a continuation of emotional support from both their mothers and fathers throughout childhood.

Adaptation to these pressures can lead boys to solve problems and express all kinds of emotions more through action than words, in contrast to girls. Some propose differences in rates of biological development between girls and boys (Kindlon & Thompson 1999). Higher activity levels, lower impulse control and slower development of fine motor skills are said to lead to later maturity in the cognitive milestones such as colour recognition, language, reading and counting. Whether it is the result of biology or adaption, boys and girls do tend to develop different 'styles' early in life. Greater sensitivity and flexibility by parents, child-care centres and elementary schools to the 'style' of boys, and to their readiness for structured learning is needed to prevent boys 'tuning out' or 'turning off' because of feelings of failure to meet expectations. Protection by caregivers and institutions from the peer bullying and pressure to conform to masculine myths, is also important for boys throughout childhood and adolescence.

NEW MODELS FOR FATHERING

If men are to become more involved, empathic fathers and positive role models for children, opportunities are needed for men to learn about what children need for survival and development. While new fathers are often encouraged to participate in the birth of the child, taking on a role of primary or equal care of an infant requires real determination, as subtle signals from peers, other family members and the mother may nudge men into a back-up role.

Is there any evidence to say that men cannot become very appropriate attachment figures for babies? As mentioned, Bowlby assumed that mothers should be the primary attachment figure for infants. Current child development theorists still propose that infants are born with attachment behaviours designed to increase their proximity to care and protection and improve their survival chances. However, the person to whom the baby attaches does not necessarily have to be the infant's mother, nor does it have to be a woman. Babies can attach to any person who spends time with them and who has the opportunity and capacity to develop a reciprocal relationship of nurture and interaction (Belsky & Cassidy 1996).

For men, just as for women, experiencing the total responsibility for attending to the hourly needs of a young baby really concentrates learning about what needs to be done. Bonding occurs through the baby's smiling, copying and preferring them to others. If such bonding develops, deliberate harm to the baby or child becomes much less likely. Therefore, the opportunity for men to directly care for infant children can be one positive way to change men's attitudes, relationships and behaviours. As mentioned earlier, a strong proviso for the safety of the babies, is that such contact occur in safe, supported environments and that inexperienced, personally needy men are not lumbered with this responsibility unprepared.

The current construction of masculinity tends to constrain men's interaction with children as they grow through the pre-teen years in a number of ways. For example, many men find surrendering the immediate control and direction of play activity and participating in imaginary games difficult because of their own socialisation to be in control. Thus they often return to a teaching role, reducing the opportunity for emotional closeness. Playing with children, letting down some of those defences, is something many men have to learn anew.

The need to be in control also colours men's attitude to discipline, seeing it more often as learned through punishment, physical hurt or endurance, especially for boys. Positive approaches (rewards, discussion, choices) to teach self-discipline are also likely to create closer relationships between the discipliner and child (Francis *et al.* 1995).

Another important issue that children need men to reconsider is physical touch and display of affection. Few people would argue that an affectionate touch or hug conveys an extra dimension of emotion and care, and for children it strengthens self-esteem and a sense of belonging. Boys in particular are deprived of this for fear they will become effeminate. This may have contributed to many men finding it hard to express affection in a physical way to anyone, but also to their lacking the ability to distinguish between affection and sexuality—affectionate touches and sexual touches. Through adults giving and explicitly teaching non-sexual touching, children learn to get intimacy needs with adults met without sexuality, until that becomes appropriate in adolescence. It is also important men assume the responsibility to recognise if sexual feelings are aroused by the touch of others and to behave appropriately around children. Certainly, men need more safe opportunities in which to discuss these sensitive issues in order to become more aware and comfortable with them. If men wish to be involved in caring for children it is necessary for them to be proactive in creating such opportunities.

ADVOCACY FOR CHILDREN AT A SOCIAL LEVEL

If men consider their own and others' children important they can seek to demonstrate this publicly by the personal and professional choices they make and the issues they support. While individual men may make decisions to spend time with children, our society does little to assist working men to do so, or to be connected into their schooling, child care, and recreational activities. Advocacy is needed, by men joining with women, to get businesses, politicians and public institutions to make children's needs a higher priority. Fathers making children more visible in their working lives might be one option, through father and child days at work or fighting for government incentives to corporations who provide or assist with child care. Fathers taking the initiative to be more involved in their children's lives is another, such as asking for information/discussion opportunities at schools, child-care centres, hospitals, community and adult education centres. Funding for some of these positive efforts will be easier to obtain than funding for child protection.

It is often difficult for institutions to engage men in reflection and discussion about children. Books have appeared in recent years in which men review their own relationships with their fathers (for example, Williams 1996). These provide an opportunity for some men to reflect in private about their own experiences before entering public discussion of issues between fathers and children with less embarrassment. Innovative approaches through other media are needed to engage non-readers in reflection on their attitudes towards their fathers.

It is important that promoting opportunities for men and fathers to be more involved with children is not done at the expense of mothers who already are. As has been stated earlier, the best situation for children results when fathers add their nurturing care to that given by mothers, not substitute for it, and when men and women both remain in emotional contact with children. Ideally men will become active in advocating for policies and programs that provide a cooperative community, supporting and protecting children from abuse and violence.

CHILD PROTECTION POLICIES AND MEN

A 'knee jerk' reaction from child protection policies that is limited to preventing men in the community from contact with children seems counterproductive if the end goal is better relationships between men and children. Policies can be developed to encourage men working with and caring for children, if the concerns are made explicit and the safeguards obvious. For example, pairing and mentoring old trusted staff and volunteers with new ones in child protection agencies, child-care centres, schools and foster agencies can protect the men from anxiety and allegations as well as the children. Men employed to work with children have to be emotionally mature enough to recognise the issue and swallow any initial defensive reaction.

Child protection policies and the agencies themselves have been notorious for ignoring men in their direct work with families of reported children, from the initial referral, through investigation, case conferencing and implementation of care plans (O'Hagan 1997). So often it is the mother of the children on whom expectations of improved care are placed, yet the father may have as much or more influence on success and less idea how to go about it. Workers ignore the male family member through fear, practical difficulties in contacting him, assumptions about gender roles, general hostility to men, or lack of training and agency support. As O'Hagan (1997) says, in some cases it is not appropriate to include dangerous men in these processes, but in others, failing to do so limits the long-term effectiveness of change for the child. It also may model inability to resolve conflict, or powerlessness in the face of an abuser to the child and other family members.

Child protection agencies and their staff need to continually review their attitudes and assumptions, as well as their training and staff support mechanisms in order to deliver equality of engagement and treatment of men and women staff, volunteers and clients. In investigation of child protection reports, the information gathered should be primary in reaching conclusions, rather than gendered assumptions. If investigators can deal honestly with hostility or a challenge of bias from an accused man, there is a much greater chance of developing a working relationship to improve a child's situation. For these reasons it is very useful in any child abuse investigation teams to have both men and women involved, providing a balance for the investigators and the investigated. It is unwise to assume, however, that in male/female teams, male workers should provide 'protection' for female ones in intimidating situations. This masculine stereotyping puts pressure on male workers to suppress any anxiety and may lead to poor decision-making by all.

For child abuse prevention, the continuation of public education efforts about child abuse, child-rearing and child development are also important. Targeting this educational material more at men and in public and work environments rather than in the home would be useful. The collection and objective analysis of statistics on reports of child abuse and their investigation and outcomes is also part of this public education. Being clearer about who hurts children and why, enables services to be better targeted, yet also avoids exaggeration of the dangers through lack of accurate information. The publication of these statistics needs to be accompanied by commentaries that discuss some of the underlying issues raised. Links with men in the media need to be developed to make men's relationships with children a 'mainstream' topic.

Also of crucial importance is support and therapy for the abused child and family, and for the abuser, in whatever professional and non-professional combinations are most appropriate to the individual situation. Helping abused children recover, and preventing adults from re-abusing, are powerful tools in overall prevention.

MEN IN CHILD PROTECTION WORK

Men who continue to work in child protection are very special people. They have taken on a role that is unusual and against the masculine stereotype of 'suitable' male professions. By this very choice they are making a statement of the value of children. They are daily faced with the distressing effects of abuse of children by others of their own sex, more so than women in the field, leading to personal questions about the nature of men and where they fit within that. They have the extra burden of dealing with anti-male sentiment from many victims, parents and female co-workers. Child protection work also often requires hearing about the sexual abuse of children. Men and women workers have to be very aware of their own feelings and responses to this; hearing the stories can affect their personal sexual identities and relationships. All these pressures mean men working in child protection have to be better than most men at recognising, confronting and resolving their own responses and emotions on a daily basis, in order to survive and be effective in their work.

Such men can provide wonderful role models to the children and adults they see in their work. Some parents of children abused by men, particularly those sexually abused, assume that the child will not want to be in contact with a male child protection worker or therapist. Sometimes this is the case, but more often the children are quite able to distinguish a caring man who is sensitive to their needs and the experience of being safe in his company is a powerful therapeutic gift.

It is also important that men are available as counsellors and therapists of other men, whether they are men who have been abusive or fathers trying to deal with the abuse of their child. The subjects of violence and sexuality can be very difficult to discuss across gender. A different kind of collegial counselling relationship may be able to develop between same-sex participants.

Men working in social welfare agencies are increasingly rising into supervisory and managerial positions, because of their career expectations, their greater opportunity to work fulltime and longer hours and their greater comfort with the current management ethos. As managers, it is incumbent on them to promote policies of anti-oppression, respect and care within their agency as well as within their practice field. Also, while it is good to have men's input into child protection policy development, ideally some experienced male child protection workers will remain at the interface working with the children and families to continue to model how men can care for children.

10 | Pitfalls and challenges in work with men who use violence against their partners

Rob Hall

In my work with men who have abused women, I have four central themes: safety, responsibility, accountability and respect (Colley *et al.* 1997). I did not develop these themes by myself. Neither was my exploration of their meaning and applicability to practice an isolated one. However, the way these themes have developed in my work and life, and the way they support and weave connections with each other, is the background to the work I do with men who have abused. This chapter is an exploration of my relationship with these themes, and the dilemmas they raise.

It is intriguing to reflect that, like many graduates, my first position as a social worker was dealing with abuse and family violence. However, the postgraduate course I had completed did not explore the dilemmas or complexity of the issues faced by most social workers in the field. I found I was in a position where my qualification did not equip me to deal with issues of abuse and power.

In the 1970s a number of South Australian women had drawn attention to the fact that women were more at risk of abuse and assault from the men they were married to, or lived with, rather than from strangers. They demanded that the community place real value on the safety of women in their own homes (Women's Information Switchboard 1980). Women started providing specialist services for women, in the health sector, the home and the workplace, and these services were aimed at addressing issues of safety. They asserted that the community should fund these gender-specific services, and they started to have some success. At this time women had very little reason to trust men working in the field of abuse, and good reason to fear that tentative gains in community funding would easily be eroded or withdrawn.

When I first started to work in the area of domestic violence, I was aware of the contribution feminist thought had made to my life and relationships. Other men and women, and myself, believed that feminist approaches could assist both men and women. We worked and consulted with each other to deal with the complexities involved in working with men's violence towards women. The dilemmas we faced have not lost their relevance, although the politics may appear to have changed. This chapter explores these dilemmas and the principles that have been helpful in dealing with them.

RESPONSIBILITY

I first began to consider the principle of responsibility in 1980 when I worked at the Crisis Care Unit, which was then a 24-hour call-out counselling service. This service was established with the support of the South Australian police, partly in the hope that it would help them to respond better to 'domestics'. The story, in common circulation at that time, was that the police were tired of revisiting the same houses in an attempt to try to 'settle domestic disturbances'. Although the issue was about the safety and protection of women, the police did not regard 'domestics' as 'real' police work. They hoped that counselling would solve the problem. Crisis Care focused its intervention on helping women to 'escape'. By doing so, the Unit and the community had clearly started to make the safety of women and children a priority, and developed a deep respect for the work and role of women's shelters.

Men, however, were rarely charged with assault, and at that time there was no legal protection through 'restraint' or 'domestic violence orders'. The Crisis Care workers believed their only role was to help women and children to get to a safe place where others understood what they were going through. Shelters were the only focus of intervention.

A group of Crisis Care workers eventually decided to examine the issues being raised by their clients. It is not surprising that this group was comprised mostly of female workers. It became clear that the women subjected to abuse were being left to carry the burden for all family members. They were taken to safe houses with security screens on every window. They were asked to relocate their children into new schools and even expected to work out solutions to end their partner's violence. No one asked, or even expected, men to take responsibility for their abusive behaviour towards their families. There were no legal or social sanctions for men who abused and no services that might expect or assist these men to take responsibility for their actions.

We faced several challenges at the Crisis Care service in 1980. How could we provide services for men that assisted them to take responsibility for abusive actions without:

- threatening funding for women and women's services;
- compromising the safety of women and children; or
- providing a soft option to the criminal justice system?

This challenge led to the commencement of work with men conducted in consultation with women's services and which attempted to be accountable and not an alternative to the criminal justice system.

We soon discovered pitfalls in these early services for men. Some of these came from workers holding an extremely narrow view of responsibility, which did not extend far beyond requiring men to face the legal consequences of their actions.

Such a limited view of responsibility did not help the men appreciate the full nature, meaning and consequences of their abusive actions. It did not challenge the common but unhelpful stand of minimisation. A working definition of responsibility needed to be broad enough to include the man facing the fact that he had abused the people he claimed he loved most. We began to face the practical challenge of finding a way to help men take full responsibility for their violence and abuse.

Having come from a lecturing environment and being familiar with feminist ideals, I had a strong, self-righteous propensity to lecture the men I was counselling. I would argue strongly for the man to address his abuse, only to find that he would argue equally strongly to justify or minimise his actions. In addressing this issue Alan Jenkins (1990) used the term 'invitation' to illustrate a process by which men might be invited to take up arguments for responsibility, respect and for non-abusive ways of being a man. This more comprehensive understanding of responsibility, incorporating practices as well as objectives, led to furthering an understanding of how the man might take full responsibility for his violence and abuse.

The criminal justice system still faces an enormous challenge in facilitating men taking full responsibility for abusive behaviour. Too often, men who wish to take full responsibility and face the consequences of their actions find themselves in conflict with their own lawyers, who believe that they are working for the best interests of their clients by encouraging the man to deny, minimise or excuse his behaviour. They see it as their responsibility, in an adversarial system, to refute the evidence of the prosecution or to argue mitigating circumstances. I have had a number of clients argue for honesty and struggle to find ways to give their lawyers instruction that they want to plead guilty.

A challenge for the criminal justice system is to adopt criteria for sentencing that relate to a definition of responsibility that encompasses more than just attending counselling. It would be helpful for the court to take less interest in mitigation of responsibility, and more interest in an assessment of the extent to which the man is taking responsibility for the abuse he perpetrated.

In helping men to undertake a journey of facing responsibility, we must negotiate the pitfall of only 'joining with' them rather than assisting them to face responsibility. If my attempts to be respectful and encouraging of the man do not include inviting him to challenge his irresponsible ideas and practices, then I fail to promote responsibility. Furthermore, I must watch the language that I use and avoid talking about his partner in objectifying terms, such as referring to her as 'she' rather than using her name. This helps to ensure that partners are always regarded as a real person in our conversations.

ACCOUNTABILITY

The principle of accountability, as developed by Tamasese and Waldergrave (1994), has helped in facing the challenge of making this work truly respectful of women's and children's experiences. It is a principle that provides helpful guidance in exploring a common difficulty even for experienced counsellors, that of helping a man with the issue of facing up. An example counsellors have shared with me is of a man in a group who gives a responsible and remorseful account of an abusive incident. The man's affect seems appropriate to his story of the incident. The counsellor believes he should appreciate what the man is doing, praise him and encourage him in setting an example for the others in the group. At the same time, it is easy to fail to give due consideration to what the abuse had meant for his partner and children and privilege his experience over their's. Invariably the counsellor who contacted his partner would learn he had a lot more facing up to do. His remorseful account is just the beginning of the more detailed exploration into understanding the extent and effects of the abuse upon his partner and children. The challenge was, and still is, how do we establish practices that hold our work accountable to the experiences of women and children who have been subjected to abuse?

Accountability practices have considerable impact on the nature of the work. To illustrate this, I will relate a set of circumstances in a men's group that I ran at the time this idea was first being explored. Letters were sent out to women partners informing them of the man's attendance at the group. We attempted to get first-hand experience of how these letters might be received through a consultation with a group of women survivors and activists known as WOWSafe (Women of the West for Safe Families). One of these women had received our letter. She explained that she was disappointed, angry and found the letter extremely intrusive when she first received it. On reading the letter more closely, she realised that she knew one of the leaders running the group and decided to contact him. She made it very clear that she had not been in a relationship with this man for at least two years. He clearly was not respectful of his ex-partner's termination of the relationship. This feedback made a major difference to our work with the man and the way in which we talked with him about his view of the relationship.

Accountability practices have major benefits for the safety of women and children. For example, a men's group worker who made contact with a woman partner discovered that she had been beaten by her partner after a group meeting. The worker was then able to put her in contact with women's services who found a safe place at a secret location. The significance of safety should never be overlooked.

The women of WOWSafe drew attention to a potential difficulty when men attend therapy or a men's group. The men's partners may develop unrealistic hopes, based on his attendance alone, that this time he will change. These hopes can override their own judgments and lead them to stop paying attention to their own experience of their partner's behaviour. Women may then make judgments about staying in relationships longer than is safe. Accountability to women's experience requires that the men's group worker must be realistic about the influence of men's groups and not overstate their effectiveness.

So, how do we access the experience of women and children without implying that they are responsible for men's abusive behaviour, or that they have any responsibility for changing or monitoring men's behaviour, or compromising their safety or wellbeing?

Another pitfall with established men's programs stems from the failure to make accountability to women's experience a priority and therefore a failure to provide adequate resources. Accountability practices require men's group leaders to make contact with women partners or an advocate (where appropriate). These practices require another form of accountability to women's services so that the work is held transparent and open to ongoing critique and development. Accountability practices are fundamental for maintaining the relevance of this work in challenging a society that promotes men's power over women.

PARTNERSHIP

Another guiding concept is partnership between service providers for services for men and for services for women. Partnership requires those working with men and those in women's groups working together for the same common goal, appreciating and respecting the different roles and responsibilities in the work, while fostering a relationship based on trust and genuine accountability. The South Australian Competency Standards for Intervention Workers, *Working with Men who Perpetuate Domestic Violence and Abuse* (1999) and the *Stopping Violence Groups* handbook (1997) are examples of successful collaboration between those working with men who have abused, women working with women and women activists.

In the 1980s men's workers assumed that the notion of men taking responsibility required this work should only be conducted by men without reference to women. This notion led to several problems:

- the unique and vital contribution of women and their place in the work tended to be discounted;
- critical feedback by women was not sought; and
- women's experience was not accorded importance or status in the work.

It is important to acknowledge the feminist roots of this work. Some agencies have disregarded the need for an accountable profeminist approach. Some have accorded greater financial and organisational status to men who work with males who abuse while women who work with women may find their work taken for granted.

The history of work with men has derived from the approaches and principles developed in the women's movement. The early pioneering work and struggle by women is too often taken for granted. In South Australia, a number of women's services, in their initial struggle to fund shelters, found the courage to go to the front bars of hotels to ask men for financial help. Front bars were traditionally part of the culture that supported men's power over women as being a 'natural' right.

The notion that work with men is men's business only led to a further difficulty whereby the value of women as co-leaders of men's groups was overlooked. In South Australia a number of women have chosen to be involved with services for men (Colley 1991). The practice of having women lead groups with men has become increasingly common in South Australia, to the extent where its benefits are now believed to be self-evident. When two group leaders of different gender relate in ways that are respectful and equitable, the very day-to-day structure and operation of the group provides a direct and visible challenge to the gendered power imbalances of the dominant culture in our society.

Men, who have attended stopping violence groups, have remarked on the benefits of mixed gender group leadership, which include:

- a sense of confidence that the woman's view would be represented throughout the program;
- a belief that a woman would be able to ask questions and present viewpoints that were informed by women's experience; and
- the belief that a woman co-leader would be in touch with the 'way we had hurt our partners' and would 'help us to look

deeper' at the effects of violence upon family members (Northern Metropolitan Community Health Service 1997, p. 58).

However, a co-working relationship that was reflective of or typified the traditional gender power imbalance would be problematic. For example, in a co-leader relationship where the female leader was a young student with little experience and the male was older and more experienced there is potential for a traditional power imbalance to be reflected in their working relationship. There is an illustrative anecdote where a young woman in her first men's group had little interaction in the group but was given the job of organising the teas and coffees and ensuring that the whiteboard was clean. Such a relationship does not propose an alternative to dominant culture. It is essential to find a way of working that highlights and deals with the complexity of the relationship between the co-leaders of different gender. A partnership between co-leaders should not expect women to join in this work nor reduce the responsibility of men for examining and challenging their gendered ways of working.

It is an ongoing challenge to find ways to ensure that the co-leader relationship is one of partnership that promotes gender accountability and respectful ways of relating between men and women.

RESPECT

In work with men who have abused, a prime objective is to foster respectful ways of relating to women. The principle of respect has played an important role in informing many aspects of the work with men. One aspect invites reflecting on the practices of intervention. For example, in my therapy how could I reasonably expect men to adopt respectful ways of relating to others if I did not relate to them with respect? Fundamental to respectful practices is the consideration of how we maintain a position of respect towards the man we are counselling, without condoning his violence and abuse and remain accountable to the experience of those he has abused.

It is most important not to lose sight of the impact and hurt that a man's actions and attitudes have imposed upon his partner and children, despite the high level of distress necessarily associated with this knowledge. My level of distress and outrage increases when the man appears to be preoccupied with self-centred attempts to minimise or discount the experiences of those he has hurt. Despite this I have an obligation to maintain a position where I respect the steps that he is taking towards responsibility and respectful ways of relating. Only then can I assist him to find the courage and motivation to face the shame of what he has done as he begins to appreciate the full meaning and impact of the abuse he has perpetrated.

Among the complexities faced in counselling are:

• how do we help him to find that emotional or mental space, which enables him to face the full meaning and impact of his abusive actions; and
• how do we help him to realise the significance of the hurt he has caused to those he loves in a way that enables personal responsibility but avoids self-deprecation?

To meet these challenges men are invited to identify their ethical and honourable life goals and intentions they have held for their positions as partners and fathers. They are invited to consider how much they have betrayed their own goals, to realise they have been capable of hurting those they love and to face the significance and extent of the damaging effects of their actions on the lives of their children and partner. To appreciate this, without a context of honour and self-respect through responsibility and facing shame, can invite men into a place where they feel overwhelmed with depression and guilt.

The process undertaken by a couple who were reconciling is illustrative. The man had completed a stopping violence group. He appreciated his abuse of her was totally his problem. His partner was asking him to understand fully what his violence and abuse had meant to her. She could not trust him nor reconcile until she felt sure that he had a thorough grasp of the meaning and effects of his abuse on her. She believed it was his job to come to these realisations himself, without her involvement. The process and its outcome, however, needed to be accountable to her experience. They jointly agreed on a meeting where he would read out and offer her a statement of realisation that he had previously prepared separately.

To achieve these realisations, he was required to revisit all abusive incidents. This required homework, considering and doc-umenting the times and ways he had hurt her and imagining her experience. He was set questions such as:

- What would it have been like for Jane to live with the level of uncertainty about her safety and to appreciate the threat was coming from you?
- What would your violence and abuse have been saying to Jane about how you see her as a person?
- As a mother, what would Jane's concerns have been for her daughters?
- What would your stepdaughters, Sue and Heather, have experienced?
- After your abuse of Jane—their mother—how might Sue and Heather regard boys and men in their lives?

He worked on these issues over time, shared his understandings and faced further questions, which we generated as we worked to understand the impact of the abuse he had chosen to inflict on Jane. He felt ashamed of his behaviour. He felt grief and deep sorrow for the hurt he had caused and for the lasting impact of his violence. Along with these realisations, he appreciated he was moving towards a position of not tolerating violence and abuse as a way of life. He was adopting practices that were respectful and considerate of others. Through his journey he was becoming the partner and stepfather he wanted to be.

His statement of realisation consisted of only a few pages. However, he had taken no shortcuts in doing the work that was needed to make that statement meaningful. On inviting his partner to witness his statement of realisation, we made it clear that she could choose the time, manner and place so this was to happen at her pace and in a way that she would feel most comfortable with. We supported her choosing the location, having someone to support her or to decline the invitation if she chose. She chose to continue with the process.

A potential pitfall is faced when couples come together and men take steps to demonstrate their responsibility. Women partners may feel an expectation to forgive and put their experience of past abuse behind them. Men may believe that past abuse should be forgotten. This couple remained very clear—in order for lessons to be learned and for the relationship to be placed on a new footing, those instances could never be forgotten. They were aware that this was only a small part of an ongoing journey of learning.

Workers face a challenge to find appropriate assessment tools to measure and monitor levels of respect, accountability and responsibility throughout the journeys undertaken by their clients.

Outcome measures and evaluation tools should contribute to the journey and to be appropriate they need to:

- have a solution focus, while assessing levels of responsibility and respectful behaviour;
- be able to be administered respectfully and collaboratively;
- assist the man to monitor his own progress towards his goals; and
- highlight new directions or options for further respectful actions.

Alan Jenkins has been working on just such a tool that can be used in collaboration with men and the people close to them. The assessment becomes a part of a continuous journey and promotes the discovery of respectful ways of being rather than a static form of assessment at the end of counselling (Northern Metropolitan Community Health Service 1997, pp. 171–99).

A significant complexity is taking account of men's own experience of abuse and injustice. Our acknowledgment of the hurt and injustice they have faced can potentially invite men to abdicate responsibility for their own behaviour. Men who have been abused by their fathers sometimes offer this as a causal explanation and excuse for their abusive behaviour. However, it is clearly unjust to ignore men's experience of abuse yet expect them to face up to the effects of the abuse they have perpetrated.

The challenge we face is how to acknowledge a man's experience of injustice without sacrificing responsibility and appreciation of the injustice that he has perpetrated.

CONCLUSION

In conclusion, I want to share my own ongoing personal challenge that I work with constantly. How can I continue to move this work in a direction of respect, responsibility, accountability, taking account of safety, and do this in partnership with those most affected by this issue?

Some practices I have adopted in response to this complexity include:

- Making direct contact with those who have been hurt or their advocates. This requires sensitivity to the fact that this may not be appropriate, in so far that the contact could be too intrusive, the person too young or they have no further interest in the matter.

- I try to imagine what it might be like for the person who was hurt to hear the conversation I am having with the man. How might they feel about what they are hearing and seeing? How might they regard the way in which the issues are being dealt with? The way their experiences are being discussed and the direction that the counselling is going?

The longer I do this work and the more people I have consulted, the more I am aware of the challenges and pitfalls of work with men who have abused. Some of these issues are part of a societal response and some are organisational responses. At times the hardest of these to deal with, and to be aware of, are those that come from the culture of masculinity that are reflected in my own attitudes. I continue to seek ways to challenge those areas in myself.

11 | Restorative justice conferencing: Reconstructing practice with male juvenile offenders

Mark Griffiths

The purpose of this chapter is to examine the challenges of working with young males in the juvenile justice system. Young males predominate in the criminal justice systems and yet there has been very little examination of the influence of masculinity on offending. To illustrate how masculinity affects juvenile crime, I will share my experiences in juvenile justice, using a typical case example of a young man found guilty of numerous house burglaries. A restorative justice group conference was held to assist the Children's Court in sentencing him. The case illustrates how restorative justice conferences can challenge the dominant traditional masculine discourse in juvenile justice.

JUVENILE JUSTICE AS A MALE-DOMINATED WORK DOMAIN

Previously, juvenile justice was dominated by institutional care as the dominant service response to juvenile crime. Institutional centres for young male offenders were centres of hegemonic masculinity. Male working-class, union-oriented youth officers dominated the service arena. There were legendary stories of senior youth officers who were powerful figures commanding enormous respect and authority in handling the most difficult and violent young men our society could produce. Senior welfare department male managers experienced their rites of passage in direct management of these institutions.

The rise of the mega-departments of health and human services, the managerial revolution and feminist public policy have changed the work domain of juvenile justice. Challenges to male hegemony in juvenile justice include the rise of women in senior management (Mahdi *et al.* 1987) and the propensity for large mega-departments of human services to regular periods of downsizing and restructuring of workplaces.

Male-dominated unions gradually lost control of worksites, resulting in more flexible working conditions and the patriarchal power of male youth officers was seen as regressive and harmful for male clients. Many male staff have found these changes very challenging and negative. Despite these changes, men in juvenile justice have rarely considered their role as men and the gender needs of other male staff and their clients until very recent times.

Men in juvenile justice are beginning to address these issues. Initially much anger, resentment, suspicion and fear has been expressed inside and outside the bureaucracy about these early, often faltering, attempts to discuss these issues. Without careful consideration and deep reflection on the beneficial aspects of the changes emerging in juvenile justice, there is always the risk that dialogue among men reverts to traditional male posturing and attempts to maintain juvenile justice as a male preserve. Men are only beginning to understand that global changes require a deep change to their own perception of themselves as well as the learning of new skills and roles. The human possibilities for an emancipatory practice are developing among male youth workers willing to accept the challenge to reinvent themselves.

Although young male offenders are the predominant clients of juvenile justice, gender issues are rarely considered. For example, masculinity is not acknowledged as a risk factor in developing primary prevention strategies. Risk-taking, non-involvement in domestic life, superficial mateship, male honour, toughness, emotional invulnerability and sexually predatory behaviours are all 'normal' male precepts that influence and shape the meaning and form of the male offending. Challenging young men's perceptions of appropriate masculinity and their offending actions also requires male juvenile justice workers to question their own models of work and self-image of masculinity (Hudson 1988).

THE DOMINANT DISCOURSE IN JUVENILE JUSTICE

The dominant discourse in current Western juvenile justice systems is based upon bureaucratic-instrumental reasoning. Technological progress and refinement of the existing technologies such as improved case management practices are promoted. As government spending increases are marginal, at best, the emphasis in state-managed justice systems is on better targeting of programs based upon a perceived 'objective' process of gathering evidence-based empirical data to guide policy and practice refinements. It is argued that more precision will produce better products (McGuire 1995).

In the front line of practice, there are practitioners who are able to temper the excessive demands of the bureaucratic system. These practitioners spend considerable time with young men and women under supervision despite the excessive paperwork and computer assisted reports that must be written for the range of administrative and judicial bodies.

The dominant discourse in Western juvenile justice systems is exemplified by the modern office accommodation where clients are seen, and the modern secure units with advanced security systems that house only the highest risk offenders in short stay facilities where 'comprehensive program planning' is undertaken. Young offenders and their families are rarely engaged in garages, train stations, camping trips and at home.

The emphasis is on control, efficiency, risk management and good public relations. Victims are not seen as proper clients of the system. Other victim support services are funded to assist them. Their interests are viewed as in opposition to the offenders' needs.

The family of the offender and surrounding community are rarely involved in this model. The juvenile justice worker will have a case load of twelve high-risk offenders, many of whom are very unreliable in reporting as directed on a weekly basis to the office as required by their statutory orders. The worker may have two urgent court reports to complete on current cases who are returning to court for reappearances. A pre-court report may need to be written within the week on a new offender and the parole board wants a report done on a young person due for release next week. What gets priority here in addition to the other normal staff meetings and supervision and staff training requirements of the job? Seeing clients for office-based reporting interviews is a core bureaucratic responsibility. Writing reports for external bodies and case management reports are all highly visible accountable instrumental outputs of the current system.

Is it not difficult to understand why workers cannot reach out to the extended family networks of young offenders to help them create the informal control arrangements that would really make a difference. As a juvenile justice worker has never met any of the victims of the young offenders, they can have little real understanding of the community harm that has been caused by juvenile offending. The worker may be unaware of the bias in practice that minimises the accountability of young offenders for the impact of their offending. So the primary objective of working with the young offender becomes to get the young person through the period of the sentencing order.

There is little known about the outcomes of the existing model of juvenile justice. Direct service workers who want to engage young clients and really assist them complain that they are spending increasing time in front of their computers. There is a false technocratic assumption that it is the right intervention of the system that will minimise an offender's criminal career.

The primary responsibility of the juvenile justice worker could be defined as communication and engagement with the people most affected by juvenile crime. 'Out of office' work would be the primary mechanism of engaging people in the communities. A new paradigm such as restorative justice challenges our whole approach to young male offenders.

THE RESTORATIVE JUSTICE CHALLENGE

Restorative justice is concerned with the community of interest created by the harmful impact of crime and faces the resultant disorder created in the social setting. It is concerned with healing the harm caused by crime, so the system accepts more responsibility for other clients, victims and the community affected by crime. In the process it reinvents its objectives and changes the roles and responsibilities of the juvenile justice worker. Restorative justice has been defined as 'any program that encourages the victim and offender to negotiate an agreement to repair the harm done' (MaCold 1997). At its core, it provides for active participation by those most affected by the offences.

Crime harms offenders far more than they realise and helping offenders gain this awareness is one of the primary aims of the restorative system. Offenders never seem to make connections between the harm, suffering and inconvenience they cause others and the direct consequences of crime on themselves and other less direct impacts such as their 'bad luck, and lack of opportunities'. Most offenders are not sufficiently stable, insightful or mature enough to take full responsibility for the impact of their offending. Restorative justice brings this challenge into their lives (Bazemore & Walgrove 1999).

Restorative justice is often described as a middle way between the current offender-focused, minimum intervention existing criminal justice systems and the emerging retribution or mandatory sentencing 'get tough' approach with its focus on the expectations of the community and victims for harsher sentencing outcomes. It is a 'bottom-up' peacemaking and community-orientated approach to healing the conflicts that create offending. It is not a panacea for the root causes of crime but it does re-engage the community in a meaningful way that may lead communities to devise more lasting solutions. One aspect of restorative justice that rarely gets attention is the benefit for the young offender. Pepinsky (1998, p. 169) says that taking responsibility for the impact of their crimes

> allows young people who otherwise would be stereotyped as part of a criminal element to individuate themselves, to defy stereotypes, and to assume roles as responsible community members who help define what our problems with them are and breaks our addiction to trying to set wayward youth straight as we purport to be doing.

Restorative justice is also perceived as a vehicle for revitalising community corrections as a movement that emerged in the 1970s and taking it beyond the narrow confines of its focus exclusively on the offenders' needs and requirements. Offenders are community members often representing the group most excluded from mainstream community opportunities. A primary focus on challenging offenders may actually maintain and increase the social exclusion experienced by offenders. Failing to address the community factors contributing to their offending behaviour, such as unemployment and poor skills training, can lead to adoption of a self-fulfilling prophecy, a committed anti-social offender. Restorative justice recognises that no community correctional system can restore offenders. It requires a real partnership and ownership by the community to solving crime problems and this can only be activated when the correctional system opens itself up in a pro-active participatory model involving all those people affected by crime. Restorative justice is a new paradigm for achieving some long-standing aims in community corrections.

Below is an example of restorative justice being applied to a very typical angry fifteen-year-old young man in juvenile justice with little insight and understanding of his circumstances and those of his victims.

Ben: The house burglar

The following case has been chosen because it represents many of the common practice issues faced in working with serious young male offenders.

Ben, aged fifteen years, on his second court appearance, was remanded overnight by the Children's Court after the police had charged him with six house burglaries. He was released the next day after agreeing to stringent bail conditions that included his agreement to participate in a group conference where his family, and potentially his victims, would be present.

A group conference was held and was attended by his family, his friends, and three of his victims along with Ben's legal representative, the police officer that charged Ben, and a psychologist working with a Victim Support Group.

An agreement was reached over three hours of discussion at the group conference where the personal impact of his offending on his victims and family was explored, and the circumstances that contributed to his offending were exposed and discussed. The ways in which Ben could make amends to his current victims and prevent further offending were agreed upon.

At the Children's Court, the magistrate accepted the agreement reached by the group conference and placed Ben on a Good Behaviour Bond that required no further statutory intervention, providing he followed through with the agreed plan. Ben completed the plan and never offended again.

Not all cases are as successful as the intervention with Ben. Serious young male offenders who end up requiring statutory community or custodial supervision will usually receive a series of supervisory orders over a career of offending during their adolescent and early adult years (Sampson & Lamb 1995). The criminal justice systems provide a sentencing hierarchy of responses in the hope that most of the offenders will desist over time as maturation occurs. There is a concern among criminologists that the delayed rites of passage for young males to adult roles and responsibilities is behind the gradually increasing young adult male prison numbers, the houses of 'failed male initiation' (Polk & White 1999, pp. 284–302).

Maturation and other protective factors (such as the presence of respected adults who take a significant interest in the offender) that help young male offenders desist from offending are being further delayed in Western societies. The absence of crucial rites of passage experiences (such as the first real job and significant relationship) from boyhood to manhood are contributing to the increasing rise in the young adult male population under correctional supervision. What went on before, during and after the group conference with Ben and his family enabled him to divert from the system.

Ben's life circumstances

Ben had been in a major conflict with his father at home for over the last two years. Both father and son hardly spoke to one another and lived almost separate lives under the same roof. When Ben was found to be bringing stolen property back to the outside bungalow where he now lived, his father ordered him to leave home.

So Ben went to live with some mates. Nancy, a single mother, lived at the house providing a safe haven for friends of her two sons who were in trouble at home. Her eldest son Terry, aged eighteen years, was responsible for keeping the boys in line.

Ben had no means of support and was not attending school. To support his new living arrangements, he committed six house burglaries, stealing various items that he could easily sell for money.

The first challenge in working with Ben was forming a constructive healing relationship with him and his immediate family and friendship network. A successful group conference needs a supporting network of people involved in the conference who can help the young person deal with the issues and accept responsibility for his offending. This network must have credibility with the young person and the victims.

The ingredients for a successful conference require the worker to engage Ben's networks and seek their participation in spite of his protests. This was a delicate process as it could have jeopardised my relationship to Ben if I negotiated their involvement without his knowledge. A unique circumstance occurred that allowed me access to Terry, with Ben present. Terry was able to understand the importance of his and Nancy's involvement, so Ben was relieved of the burden of protecting his best mate and older peer leader.

Ben's father is a patriarchal man who sees his role as protector and provider. He agrees to attend 'to protect the family'. He is an example of what Robert Bly describes as the 'erosion of male confidence' in elders and nurturing fatherhood (cited in Mahdi *et al.* 1987). Ben spurned his father and was expelled by him. However, his rigid male code of behaviour has been learned from his father and both have emotionally dissociated from their real feelings and have trouble expressing any other feelings besides anger and frustration.

Ben's mother tried to maintain contact with her son, who stoically resisted her support. He visits home very occasionally, only when his father is absent, to see his mother and his younger sister who also attended the conference.

Ben's victims
All Ben's victims were contacted by letter with multiple choice options for voluntary involvement in the process. Three families declined involvement. One family was still very traumatised by the burglary, although all Ben had stolen from their home were some beer bottles and CDs owned by their daughter. But this home invasion had affected this family the most and they decided to invest in an expensive new security system following the burglary. They could not really afford this expense as the husband was on workers compensation payments for work-related stress. Their daughter had trouble sleeping, since the burglar had entered her room for her favourite CDs. This is a common reaction among children to home invasion of their bedroom. They wanted their story told at the conference and all they wanted back were the CDs that were loved by their daughter. Three other victims also attended the conference.

The conference
A restorative justice conference makes use of the narrative of offending to allow the participants to tell their stories. Each participant in the group conference has a unique story to tell. It is in the story telling, reflection and dialogue between participants that engagement takes place, resulting in insight into the situation and cooperation for problem-solving action. Conferences take considerable time (usually two to three hours) and participants are

provided with a safe environment in which to share their feelings and views with the common purpose of healing the harm caused by offending in a way that limits further offending.

In Ben's conference, the present victims' stories contained issues of losing precious personal items and the impact on their lives of his invasion of their privacy. In hearing about the trauma faced by the absent family, they put their own concerns aside to highlight the need for Ben to address the family's request for the replacement CDs.

In re-reading a written transcript by an independent observer to Ben's conference, I am struck by the range of discussions and the active participation of those present. Conferences engage those participants most affected by offending but who are rarely engaged by the existing criminal justice system. They are an example of a new social technology in criminal justice, as it is committed to an 'open conversation between different understandings, different vocabularies, different cultural paradigms' (Tarmas 1996).

The plan

The victims present at the meeting decided that they wanted Ben to make various woodwork items for them and that they would buy these items so that he could afford to pay for replacement CDs for the daughter of the victim who was still too traumatised to be present. The present victims set aside their right to some form of symbolic reparation after hearing about the plight of the absent victim's story. This event is what makes restorative justice conferences such a welcome addition to the criminal justice system. In my five years facilitating conferences, these small acts of human civility and kindness happen too often to be described as aberrations.

Ben followed through with most aspects of the plan. He made the woodwork items to the specifications of the victims. He attended a woodwork program once per week on work experience from his school. A voucher for replacement CDs was delivered to the victim family.

Ben is back at school and now in receipt of a training allowance enabling him to pay board to Nancy. His relationship to his family improved, with him making visits home for meals, and the tension with his father has lessened.

What stopped Ben offending?

At one stage in the conference, Ben said 'I won't re-offend because now I get the training allowance and I don't need to offend'. He was homeless and largely penniless when he committed his burglary crimes and was at high risk as an early school drop-out in a high unemployment area where the youth labour market had collapsed.

Polk and White (1999) draw attention to the role of economic adversity in producing crime and delaying traditional rites of passage for young adult males that have helped most males desist from crime. Are the structural and economic factors a sufficient explanation for Ben's offending behaviour? What stopped Ben from seeking immediate help from numerous sources that were available to him in his immediate environment?

Much of Ben's offending and difficult behaviour resulted from his need to defend his male honour. He committed the crimes alone to raise money to pay his way out of home. He fought at school and was suspended over trivial issues that slighted a female friend whom he had to defend. He protected his new friends from involvement in the conference because 'it might cause them discomfort', just as his father protected the family from him. It was only when Terry immediately saw the need for his mother and himself to attend to support Ben that he became engaged in the process of the restorative justice conference. Male honour is very real and powerful. It isolates men and harms others. The positive active leadership displayed by Terry in helping Ben created a climate for him to accept responsibility and act positively towards his family and his victims. This case illustrates the many challenges of trying to work effectively with the male code of honour that harms young men and their victims.

What role did the victims play as moral agents in restoring this young man's place in his family and community? He witnessed their capacity to put aside immediate hurts and concerns for another family hurting more. Ben was a witness to his father's male protective behaviour which he learned and enacted in his own way. The victims brought a moral imagination and energy to the conference that ignited the other participants to show the same concern for others. Ben followed through on carpentry work that was detailed and time consuming and he completed the tasks, handed them over in person and received the reward of cash for the CD voucher. This process kept the victims' role alive in his mind for weeks after the conference was held and the court appearance had faded from his view.

Can a well timed once-off restorative justice conference act as a symbolic rite of passage from an offender to non-offender status? What role does the moral imagination play in developing new patterns of behaviour in young offenders? Deep connections can be formed in the conference setting between the young offender, the victims and the families and respective communities involved. These connections stimulate the group imagination, which can result in creative problem-solving and new conviction in those involved in the process.

Ben's father seemed isolated in the conference. He actively listened but was largely ineffectual. One pays a price for male honour. Perhaps it was the best he could do to keep out of the way as things got sorted around him. Ben may have learned that there might be other moral ways to deal with conflict and impulse from the strength of Terry and Nancy and the tears of his sister and support of his mother in the conference. The conference itself can act as a vehicle for providing Ben with what Coles (1997) calls a 'deep down guiding ethical compass' that only credible, dependable and believable adults can pass on to young people. Is Ben's dark 'thief in the night' behaviour a shadow reflection of the father's unacknowledged feelings of deep rejection and isolation from his father? What price do we pay for patriarchy as fathers and sons? Can we afford to continue to ignore this tragedy?

Ben's offending was the culmination of a long period when his family was placed under enormous stress through father–son conflict. There was also the absence of any communication between Ben's family and Nancy who was officially looking after her son. This absence led to no one realising that Ben had no means of support, which was the stated reason given by him for committing the offences. Ben had created this arrangement because his male code required that he be independent of anyone's help and protective of his new family (Paulsen 1999; Pollack 1998). Did Ben's enactment of his learned male code of stoic independence create the conditions for his offending?

Ben had turned sixteen by the time of the conference and his lawyer pointed out that, at eighteen, he could face twelve months inside an adult male prison for the burglaries. Are we willing to risk no or minimal intervention in the Children's Courts, given the next scenario for male youths aged eighteen years? The juvenile justice system does no favours to young men when it fails to show them the full impact of their offending on others and minimises the consequences that are imposed on them. It has a moral responsibility to examine its contribution to the rising adult male prison population.

RESTORATIVE JUSTICE AND NEW MASCULINITIES

Restorative justice work is a challenge to young male offenders and their male workers. We are witnessing the emergence of a new paradigm in criminal justice that challenges everything connected to the rationalist masculine modern view of corrections (Bazemore & Walegrove 1999). We can see this new paradigm in the following aspects of restorative justice that challenge existing practice:

- Outcomes are not as important as the process to do the restorative work. Restorative justice allows for the hidden natural capacity of people to create and work at solutions together.
- Value is placed on participation and involvement for its own sake, creating partnerships, hearing multiple perspectives, emotional work, creativity and the symbol of the healing circle. Deeper connections are created and through this new energies are utilised and harnessed.
- Passion and the expression of true feelings connect people to their own hearts and the higher powers of the group consciousness formed in a safe environment. The value of engagement skills with all aspects of the community is re-asserted.
- Time and space are created for real reflection and deep experience of community and responsibility. Silence and space are valued and created by facilitation.

The symbolic value and healing potential of these values are not new. They have been practised millenniums ago in a range of traditional cultures. Modern feminist and therapeutic writers have espoused these values. Postmodern theorists would understand and acknowledge similar trends and changes in values across most fields of human endeavour.

Restorative justice challenges hierarchy and paternalistic power. Rigid modes of thinking become exposed and this can be threatening to some males. They have to be gently encouraged to open themselves up to new influences and thinking. A realistic understanding of people's capacity to change needs to be held in this regard. Professionals such as magistrates, the police and legal representatives are also challenged, as they are not trained to collaborate with the community and share their power. Some will embrace this change and others will oppose it. By definition, restorative justice is concerned for healing and accepting of gradual change for the better.

CONCLUSION

This chapter has examined some of the challenges and issues faced in working with young male offenders in juvenile justice. The dominant narrative in juvenile justice has evolved from a patriarchal model to the current modern bureaucratic instrumental model that espouses technocratic solutions. Male workers in juvenile justice are challenged to reinvent their practice in this environment. An example of restorative justice was used to show how new models can challenge male offending codes and the dominant discourse in juvenile justice. Prevention strategies that directly challenge out-moded male patriarchal values and provide modern rites of passage experiences for young males at risk are needed beyond what is illustrated in this chapter.

Restorative justice strategies such as group conferencing can help break down the impact of the negative and rigid male codes of conduct. The case example illustrates the use of the conference as a symbolic rite of passage for male offenders. Utilising the powers of naturally occurring communities of interest in the family, community and victims, the conference is a vehicle for learning about new ways of operating that are not harmful to others. When the offender ceases this behaviour, other benefits begin to flow towards them. It is not going to be easy for males to embrace these values and for restorative justice to reinvent juvenile justice. A significant community effort will be required. However, successful outcomes, such as the intervention with Ben, provide hope for the future.

12 | Masculinity, offending and prison-based work

David Rose

The reasons why people commit crimes are multifaceted and often debated, as are strategies to reduce crime. However, as Newburn and Stanko (1994, p. 1) conclude, 'the most significant fact about crime is that it is almost always committed by men'. This chapter first examines the nature of the relationship between men and crime and provides a brief overview of competing explanations for its existence. It also discusses other factors that impact on men who have offended, such as unemployment, educational attainment, substance misuse and men's role and place in a changing society. Some of the issues and dilemmas inherent in human service practice with this group are then focused on, with a particular reference to prison work. Finally, some practical ideas for working with men who have offended are provided, and some of the likely future developments within the field are discussed.

MASCULINITY AND CRIME

The 1999 Prison Census indicates that in Australia men make up 94 per cent of the prison population, and that almost half (49 per cent) of these men have been convicted of serious offences involving violence or threat of violence (ABS 1999). A similar trend is seen with people who have committed less serious offences and who have been placed on community-based dispositions. For example, in the state of Victoria, Australia, as at December 1999, around 83 per cent of people on community-based dispositions are men (Victorian Department of Justice 1999). International data further confirms this link between men and offending with, for example, 95 per cent of sentenced prisoners in England and Wales in 1998 being male (White 1999), and 93 per cent of prisoners in United States Federal Prisons in 1997 being male (Federal Bureau of Prisons 1997).

The relationship between masculinity and crime has long been recognised in criminological research, but paradoxically much of the research effort has been focused on attempting to explain why women offend (Buckley 1996). The 1990s saw a renewed interest in investigation of masculinity and crime against a backdrop of community and mass media concern with a perceived increasing 'crisis of masculinity'. Stanko (1994, p. 45) argues that criminology's traditional limited focus on easily observable street crime and violence has resulted in a situation which 'deflects attention away from the realities of violence in men's lives, both as perpetrators and victims'.

Stanko (1994, pp. 38–44) summarises some of the major debates that have taken place within contemporary criminology to explain the link between masculinity and crime within three broad areas. The 'nature versus nurture' debate has centred around the extent to which male violence may be a result of implicit biological factors versus the extent to which violence may be learned as young men grow up and are influenced by various institutions and factors in society. The 'instrumental versus expressive violence' debate has attempted to examine and explain the nature of violent behaviour from the point of whether the violence is intended to result in some gain (for example, instrumental violence such as a robbery to obtain material goods) or expressive violence such as a person losing their temper and resorting to violence. Finally, the 'negotiating masculinities' perspective has examined the extent to which masculine violence towards other men and women is a means of negotiating power within the hierarchies inherent in society, and as a counter-perspective to debates that attribute male violence to an individualist/socially deterministic divide (Jefferson 1994).

The 1990s have also seen the debate surrounding masculinity and crime moving with an increasing emphasis to the notions of the so-called 'problem with boys' and the associated 'crisis of masculinity' (Collier 1998). The 'crisis of masculinity' has not been limited to academic debate, and has been an issue of discussion and increasing concern within wider society and the media (*The Economist*, 28 September 1996, p. 23):

> Tomorrow's second sex: The signs are everywhere in America and Europe: more women at work; girls doing better in school; debate about 'feminisation' in America's politics; its 'million-man march'. This article summarises the evidence of a growing social problem: uneducated, unmarried, unemployed men.

Collier (1998) has documented many of the factors that appear to be contributing to this perception of a 'crisis of masculinity'. For example, there is a widespread educational failure of boys relative to girls and an increasing recognition that many young men lack the necessary personal and employment skills for modern labour markets. Family breakdown and confusion and uncertainty about the role of men in the family is apparent with an increasing concern about 'absent fathers' and the lack of role models for young men growing up in single-parent families with their mothers. Furthermore, technological advances in reproduction have further challenged traditional roles of fatherhood and resulted in media reports that men are 'redundant' in modern society. Similarly, young men are increasingly seen as either 'unmarriageable' due to their lack of employment prospects and education, or choosing not to marry and instead follow hedonistic ends.

These changes have been the backdrop for a perceived increase in violent crime and repeat offending, and a concern that there is an increasing group of young men who are uncontrollable, disenfranchised and see no useful role for themselves in a changing society (Burns 1998). Recent years have also seen far wider reporting of horrific crimes by increasingly younger men, such as killing of children or massacres, and massacres committed by lonely, disenfranchised men who are often reported to be 'paying back' society (Collier 1998). While the notion of a 'crisis in masculinity' has clearly focused attention on the relationship between masculinity and crime to unprecedented levels, it is still difficult to make any firm conclusions. As Collier suggests (1998), some of the notions implicit within the 'crisis of masculinity' thesis have been seen before (for example, the emphasis on young men from poor backgrounds), and the term masculinity itself is problematic due to its various meanings and definitions.

CONTEXTUAL FACTORS

The preceding discussion has focused on the broad theoretical explanations that seek to explain the relationship between men and crime. In undertaking work with men who have offended, it is also useful to examine a number of characteristics and factors that impact on the men and the work that is done with them. These factors may at various stages contribute to offending, or be partly a result of the offending.

Offending appears to be more highly associated with younger people, although the average age of prisoners has been increasing. In 1998 the average age of male prisoners was 33 years old with the age bracket 20–24 years old having the highest age-specific imprisonment rates in Australia (ABS 1999). A significant factor in offending is also a previous history of offences. In Australia in 1998, 63 per cent of male prisoners had previously been imprisoned under sentence (ABS 1999). Similarly, in England and Wales 53 per cent of adult males and 77 per cent of young male offenders (under 21 years old) released during 1995 were re-convicted within two years (White 1999).

Prisoners also tend to have low education levels and to have experienced high levels of unemployment. Based on data from the state of Victoria, Australia, in 1998 87 per cent of male prisoners highest level of education was part secondary with 6 per cent having completed secondary education and only 0.3 per cent having a technical or trade qualification. Furthermore, 61 per cent of male prisoners were unemployed at the time of reception into prison (OCSC 1999).

Substance misuse is a major factor in offending, with alcohol or drug use related to the offences of up to 80 per cent of the prison population (PDAC 1996). The relationship between alcohol abuse/dependence and violent behaviour is well established (NCADA 1994), as is the observation that problematic use of alcohol and/or illicit drugs is over-represented in men generally (Hall 1995). Mental illness is also over-represented in offender populations. The major study by Herrman *et al.* (1991) of the prevalence of mental illness among prisoners in Australia found that 12 per cent had a current diagnosis of mood disorder (mainly depression) and 3 per cent a psychotic disorder. Furthermore, male offenders generally are particularly vulnerable to suicide. A major review of factors impacting on suicide rates found that while being in custody increased the risk of suicide, other factors (which are common in male offenders) increased this vulnerability including being a young male, substance misuse, relationship breakdowns, unemployment and homelessness (Suicide Prevention Task Force 1997).

Offenders also tend to have significantly higher death rates than the general population. Research based on data from the state of Victoria, Australia, reveals that people in prison have a higher death rate than the general community. The death rate for offenders on community-based dispositions is even higher. The data indicates that for the 198 deaths of offenders on community-based dispositions examined, 31 per cent had died due to alcohol or drugs, and a further 15 per cent through suicide. While there were no significant differences between men and women, 86 per cent of the deaths were men, which is reflective of the proportion of male offenders (Biles *et al.* 1999).

WORKING WITH MEN IN A PRISON CONTEXT

The remainder of the chapter focuses on practice issues in undertaking human service work with this group, particularly in a prison context. My comments in this section are based on my own observations from working as a social worker with offenders in various settings and contexts. This has included mental health work in a maximum security prison, personal development groups for young male offenders on community-based dispositions, alcohol and drug assessment and treatment with offenders on community-based dispositions, and working within an agency providing post-release support to offenders in the community. The intention of this section is not to focus on specific specialist interventions but to discuss generalist work with male offenders who, as has been shown, constitute the majority of people involved with the criminal justice system. However, this is in no way intended to minimise the very significant issues that are faced by women offenders, not the least of which are the frequent lack of appropriate services because of their relatively small numbers within the criminal justice system.

Human service work with offenders clearly varies depending on the exact role the worker is undertaking. Some workers have a largely statutory role while maintaining some care functions (such as Community Corrections Officers/Parole Officers). Others perform what can primarily be seen as a caring role within a health or welfare context (such as staff providing welfare services or release preparation or therapeutic services such as alcohol and drug counselling). While the particular role of the worker varies, an underpinning goal of most human service work with offenders is to minimise their potential for further offending. The harm for victims that results following a crime is only too well known. When working with the men who have committed these offences, the significant consequences that result for themselves and their often forgotten parents, partners, children and friends also becomes only too apparent, particularly where they are serving a term of imprisonment.

Reflections on work in prisons

There can be little doubt that the prison is overwhelmingly a masculine environment. In the prison where I worked all the prisoners were men, and the majority of prison officers were men. The prison system is based, to a large extent, on the elements of discipline, control and hierarchy, both from the point of view of the officers and the structure within which they work with prisoners, and between the prisoners and the way they interact with each other. It is also an environment where violence or threat of violence or other sanctions openly mediate many of the relationships between prisoners, and in a less overt way between prisoners and staff. These factors are very common (to varying degrees) in most prisons, and as Sim (1994) argues, the overt masculine environment within prisons can be seen as a microcosm of the masculine structures that operate within society generally.

The prison system also tends to be a place of many paradoxes and contradictions that caution against viewing prisons and the people within them in a one-dimensional or stereotypical way, particularly from the aspect of human service work. For example, I was confronted early on in my work in the prison with the observation that while one of my main objectives may have been to reduce the potential for re-offending, some men did not view being in prison as necessarily an undesirable thing. While this obviously raised questions about the likely effectiveness of the work I was doing, it also raised questions about the lives some of these men were living outside the prison if it was seen as a better, and often a safer, option. Similarly, it was a regular occurrence to observe and be told of more vulnerable men who were being 'stood over' by other prisoners under the threat of violence. There was usually a very clear hierarchy among the men with certain prisoners by nature of their personal attributes or reputation and the type of offence they had committed having greater levels of power and control over others. Against this very 'macho' backdrop, however, was the fact that in working with the men I would often be presented with another perspective, such as a man crying about lost opportunities or a relationship. Similarly, particular men would sometimes demonstrate considerable concern for the welfare of another inmate.

While there are many paradoxes in working with men in prisons, there are also some common themes. What is very clear is that the majority of prisoners tend to come from very disadvantaged backgrounds. That is, many of the men I worked with had low education levels with long histories of unemployment or chaotic work history. Many had been convicted of several previous offences, often from the time of their early teenage years. Other factors such as substance abuse problems were common. A particular area of concern for many of the men was their relationships with partners, children and other family members. Where the man's offence had actually been committed against a family member this obviously had serious consequences for the particular relationship. Even when the offence was unrelated to the family member, imprisonment and further offending was often a catalyst for relationship problems and difficulties. Where the prisoner did have a supportive relationship with a family member, it was often with their mother or a female partner, and the associated absence of male family members, such as fathers, was common. Many prisoners I worked with would often describe this lack of a male role model when growing up. I was also often left with the impression that a significant number of these men had real difficulty in seeing a useful role or place for themselves in society, and would express little hope for the future.

These observations may well support notions of a 'crisis of masculinity' as some would propose, but making this exact connection is difficult and beyond the scope of this chapter. More importantly, I believe that working with these men should ensure that these factors are recognised and addressed. However, on this point, it is also important to recognise that taking account of all these factors should not result in a situation where all responsibility is removed from the man because of the oppressive situation in which they have grown up and lived and which may have contributed to their offending (Buckley 1996).

A final general point about human service work in prisons is that the role of the worker must be carefully considered. From my own perspective, I was aware that as a male social worker (often viewed as a caring, feminine profession) in a very masculine prison environment, there were real issues for the way my work was undertaken and the way I was viewed by both prisoners and prison staff. I would argue that human service staff who work with offenders in prison and in other settings must continually assess and reflect on the way they are working with the men and the effect the environment of the prison is having on their own way of working. It is not uncommon to observe human service workers in prisons who have become so entrenched in the dominant culture of the prison that, for example, they operate in a way synonymous with the correctional staff. Conversely, others have attempted to radically change or challenge systems from within with the result that their position is untenable. That is, workers need to continually aim to be offering something different from their human service perspective, while maintaining enough credibility within the dominant culture to be able to operate effectively for the benefit of the men in prison.

Key elements of human service work in prisons and following release

Based on my experience of work in a prison (providing ongoing case management and release preparation) and what operates in various prisons, some key areas that are important to address are outlined below. First, though, there are some general principles that I believe are important to guide all work with prisoners. These include:

- A holistic approach is needed that takes into account the multiple needs of the person. For example, a personal development group or men's group may be very effective but lose any real long-term benefit if the man's basic needs for accommodation, income and so on are not adequate and vice versa.
- Human service work undertaken while in prison needs to be integrated with support and services following release.
- Human service work should be undertaken in a context that is positive and gives hope for the future, and that essentially gives the person 'something to lose' by re-offending.

Within these broader frameworks, the following components can be important aspects of human service delivery in prisons:

- facilitation of family contact (where appropriate) including assisting the parties to communicate where there are difficulties and initiating contact where contact has been lost;
- interventions aimed at specific needs individuals have that impact on their offending; for example, alcohol and drug services or psycho-education groups and mental health treatment for men who have a mental illness;
- community Integration Programs that provide information on community supports and services and link the men in with these services as needed (This can also serve to provide a link for community services into the prison.);
- release preparation that ensures that necessary structures are in place following release (This includes areas such as having the required identification to access benefits, employment assistance, identification of areas for further education/training, accommodation, linkage to specialist services, and continuation of programs that have been undertaken while in prison.);
- groups or individual work that examines men's role in a changing society and how this relates to their individual experience; for example, a men's group that examines role expectations for men, the men's perceptions of women, and how these areas might relate to their current experience and offending;
- examining offending behaviour including motivation for particular offending and victim empathy; and
- general personal development such as communication skills, dealing with stress, anger management, etc.

These various components need to be provided in a coordinated way that takes account of the individual needs of the men, but that also recognises that the prison is an artificial environment for many of these activities to be taking place in, and that the real impact will only be apparent upon release. Thus it is important to link these components and any other interventions that take place in prison with what will happen following release.

My experience working in a community-based human service agency that provides support services to men following their release from prison has shown that one of the most crucial times for men who have been in prison is the initial period following release. While the men often experience considerable difficulty in re-adjusting to life in the community and gaining access to basic needs such as stable accommodation, this also takes place against a backdrop of the stigma associated with their offending and the fact that they have been in prison. It must also be recognised that release of the man from prison will often precipitate considerable stress and need for support among family and significant others. This is where progress made while in prison may be quickly lost if the man is faced with what seems like insurmountable difficulties in accessing basic needs or in relationships with others or they start to resort to their old ways of thinking or acting. Thus, I would argue that any rehabilitative component of human service work that is provided to men while in prison will only be as good as the linkages, follow-up and opportunities which are then provided in the community.

GENERAL ISSUES AND TRENDS FOR THE FUTURE IN HUMAN SERVICE WORK WITH PRISONERS

As was shown at the beginning of this chapter, the reasons why people commit crimes and why men commit the overwhelming majority of these crimes are contested. Similarly, there is considerable debate over 'what works' so far as rehabilitation of offenders and reduction of recidivism is concerned, with many people believing nothing works, and the whole area is suffering from a lack of consistent evaluation (Howells & Day 1999; Trotter 1999). However, some promising areas of potential further development for work with offenders are now outlined.

Behavioural-based rehabilitation programs

Rehabilitation programs that are behavioural-based and focus on 'criminogenic needs' have been shown to be effective in reducing offending (Howells & Day 1999). These interventions focus significantly and in a long-term way on a particular area such as substance misuse or anger management that can be directly related to the people offending. In a similar vein, the pro-social approach to working with offenders based on problem-solving and role-modelling appropriate behaviour has similar underpinnings (Trotter 1999).

Restorative justice

Restorative justice approaches such as the various community conferencing programs that have been piloted in Australia for primarily young offenders (Braithwaite & Daly 1994) are another area with promising results and the potential for greater expansion to older offenders. These programs focus on addressing the harm caused by crime through meetings or conferences and frank communication between the offender, their family, other people from the community and victims and in many models aim to divert the person from the criminal justice system.

Specialised men's groups

Programs targeting masculinity and offending such as specialised men's groups (Buckley 1996; Murphy 1996) have been effective. Given the nature of the strong link between masculinity and crime, the potential of such targeted programs is considerable, although the use of such programs has not as yet become standardised in Australian prisons.

Re-integrative programs

Programs that focus on re-integrative opportunities such as providing opportunities for housing, education and employment are also worthwhile. For example, research has shown that having a job can be one of the strongest factors protecting against further offending (Burns 1998).

Further development of effective strategies to better deal with men's violence and other offending behaviour are clearly important for assisting these men who often have backgrounds of considerable disadvantage to live more fulfilling lives. However, more important is the potential for more effective strategies to reduce the impact of offending (particularly violence) on others. This is especially so for those groups such as women and children who are often the victims of such offending and who often bear a considerable burden in supporting men who have offended (Knox 1996).

CONCLUSION

In this chapter it has been shown that while the relationship between masculinity and crime has been established, explanations for this relationship are contested. From a human service practice perspective, I have argued that men in prison often have complex, multiple needs within an overall context of structural disadvantage. Meeting some of these needs is a significant challenge for human service workers, as is the balancing role between the 'care' and 'control' functions that inevitably confront workers at the interface with the criminal justice system. Human service responses need to be multifaceted and offer a range of options and strategies, as has been outlined. These strategies need to be linked to follow-up support following release from prison to ensure they fully benefit the man in a longer-term way. It is also important that there are re-integration opportunities such as assistance with accommodation and employment that will provide the basis for the man to have a chance at a fulfilling life in the community.

PART IV

RESPONDING TO
SOCIAL DIFFERENCE
AND INEQUALITY IN
MEN'S LIVES

13 | Improving health and welfare services for older men

Fiona McDermott and
Elizabeth Ozanne

To be an older male at the present time is to have encountered and participated in profound political, social, economic and technological changes. Many of the men in the group aged 55 years and older were born during the depression of the 1930s, which impacted on their childhood years.

During late adolescence and early adulthood, the Second World War intruded upon their lives, often resulting in personal losses and psychological damage. The younger members of this cohort may have fought in the Korean and Vietnam wars, the latter in particular having been for many a traumatic, alienating and unrewarded experience.

Many of these men became fathers themselves during the 1940s and 1950s producing the 'baby boom' generation on which the economic and political aspects of their present lives now depend. The 1970s saw the emergence of 'second-wave' feminism which particularly targeted and challenged the beliefs and values concerning sexual identity, family life and gender relations with which these men had grown up and which the lives of many of them exemplified. The emergence and influence of the Gay Rights movement and increased interest in men's studies has, for the most part, ignored this older age group, except in so far as its existence may have served to challenge or disturb the status quo.

In the 1980s and 1990s the world of work, particularly for men, has been dramatically changed through the influence of globalisation, the decline of the nation state and rapidly expanding technological and communications innovations.

While older men may have in common participation in many of these historical events, recognition of their diversity remains of central importance. From within a critical theoretical perspective, the influence of gender, class and ethnicity is defining. How older men understand and interpret their lifetime experiences—their involvement or not in political processes, the importance cultural and religious institutions played in their lives, their economic and employment history, their dependency (or otherwise) on the State for health and welfare services, their experience as Indigenous Australians or as refugees or as immigrants or as belonging to a minority group—will characterise their reflections on these very experiences. As Leonard and Nichols point out (1994, p. 6) particular kinds of consciousness and subjectivity arise out of and accompany such lifetime experiences and influence older people's relations with the present, their optimism or despondency reflecting class positioning and its consequences. Indeed, economic security or its opposite is fundamental to one's capacity to be an active agent participating in shaping the social structures that constrain or enable individual and collective action.

Gender, class and ethnicity continuously interact in ways which (re)produce social relations, experiences and consciousness. However, with the process of ageing itself there is the additional factor of biological change. Advancing age brings with it organic and bodily changes, increasing frailty and the realisation of the finitude of life. Any attempt to understand older men's lives needs to place this recognition and its consequences in terms of notions of identity, subjectivity and the interpretation of need, firmly within the heuristic of class, ethnicity and gender. For example, the ways in which older men experience being cared for or being carers themselves, or access health and welfare services, or reach out to join with other community members will refer to and reflect their consciousness as subjects framed by relations of production and reproduction.

However, the task of understanding the conditions of older men's lives is confounded at the outset by social constructions which serve to obscure them, both as older persons and as males. Indeed, older people in Western liberal democracies are largely invisible and, when they are noticed, they are frequently seen in gender neutral terms and as an undifferentiated group, the diversity of whose members is ignored.

SOCIODEMOGRAPHIC PROFILE OF OLDER MEN

Mangum (1997, p. 30) in reviewing the key characteristics that locate elderly men in demographic space concluded that:

> on the negative side of the ledger, . . . they are a numerical
> minority among older persons, a fact that is reflected in a low sex
> ratio. Their life expectancy is considerably less than that of women
> of the same age as a result of their mortality rates being higher.
> Their health is somewhat poorer than that of elderly women, and
> they are much more prone to commit suicide and considerably more
> prone to die from accidents and violence. On the positive side of
> the ledger, however, elderly men are more likelier than elderly
> women to be married and living with a spouse, to have higher
> post-retirement incomes than single older women, to have more
> formal education than older women, and to have greater involvement
> in the labour force.

Although about 105 boys are born for every 100 girls, women outnumber men by age 30 because of higher male mortality rates (Mathers 1994). By age 65, the sex ratio has become highly skewed, although varying considerably across ethnic/occupational groups.

Elderly men have a much higher overall death rate than elderly women particularly from the first two leading causes of death: heart disease and cancer. The rates are not, however, uniformly higher for men and older women are considerably more likely to die from strokes and diabetes than are older men. There are hormonal, physiological and genetic differences between men and women that account for some of the variance in death rates. There are also lifestyle and workplace differences. Women are generally more health-conscious than men and differ in their health behaviours, such as seeking necessary medical care in a timelier fashion. They are also more likely to act on current advice on proper nutrition and exercise. The workplace tends to be more hazardous for men than for women because of the traditional male/female occupational structure. For instance, men have higher rates of chronic obstructive pulmonary disease because more of them smoked across the lifecourse and worked in toxic environments like coal mines, foundries and automobile paint shops. Such exposure may not catch up with them until old age.

Older persons generally have lower rates of acute conditions and higher rates of chronic conditions than do younger persons and for chronic conditions there is considerable variability by gender. Women 65 years of age and over generally have higher rates than men of arthritis, cataracts, orthopaedic impairments, diabetes, migraine and high blood pressure. Older men, by contrast, have higher rates than women of visual impairments, hearing impairments, ulcer and heart conditions. Older women have more of the chronic conditions that affect their quality of life, while older men tend to be plagued by chronic conditions that kill them.

Though suicide is not one of the seven leading causes of death among older men and women, there are large differences in suicide rates between older men and women. In Victoria in 1995, suicide rates for males aged 55 to 85 years and over far outstripped the rate for females (ABS 1997; Victorian Taskforce Report on Suicide Prevention 1997). For those aged 55–59 years there were 32 male suicides per 100 000 as compared to twelve per 100 000 for females. In the 85 years and over age group there were 48 male suicides per 100 000 compared to four per 100 000 women. In fact, in terms of rates per 100 000 population, males aged 85 years and over are the highest in all age groups although numerically this group is small. Males also have a higher incidence of deaths from accidents and violence.

Compared to single individuals of the same age, married persons generally enjoy a richer and more fulfilling social life, greater income and better health. The majority of men find themselves with a partner in late life, the majority of women without. For both elderly men and women, marital status obviously affects living arrangements. For persons 65 and over living in households, 15.5 per cent of elderly men were living alone, 41 per cent of elderly women lived by themselves.

Though the economic situation of the elderly has generally improved in the last century, there continue to be major income differentials between men and women in late life related to work history and marital status.

There are major historical deficits in the education levels of present cohorts of older persons and considerable differential between educational levels of older men and women. Though more women are currently involved in higher education this is not yet evident in late life.

There has been a long-term downward trend in employment of older males since 1900 with the phenomenon of early exit down to age 50 evident in recent restructuring economies as a consequence of both push and pull factors (Borowski 1990). Whether future labour demand will stall or reverse this downward trend is yet to be seen. Though there is some evidence for such turnaround in the US (Quinn 1999), Australian statistics continue to demonstrate a fairly persistent decrease. Older persons who are still working are usually in part-time and often low-paying jobs.

PREVAILING APPROACHES TO THE STUDY OF OLDER MEN

In the general literature the situation of older men is most often contrasted, usually negatively, to the situation of older women in that more women live on their own in late life and on a considerably smaller income and in more constrained circumstances than men. Some suggest, however, that across the lifecourse there are major points of convergence and divergence in men's and women's needs and that too great an emphasis on differentiation of the genders may be a disservice to each (Bengtson *et al.* 1996). Alternatively older men are sometimes compared to younger cohorts either in late life, for example the old old/middle old/young old, or to young or middle-aged adults. Another approach is to use a group of older men as their own control as might happen in the analysis of needs of older gay men. Each of these comparisons has particular implications in terms of what is highlighted and how service interventions might be designed to respond to perceived need.

There have been, however, some consistent lines of inquiry. In relation to the biology of older men, in an edited volume by Marie Haug *et al.* (1985) on the health and mental health status of older women, DeVore *et al.* convincingly argue the case for 'the biological superiority of women' in terms of their genetics, physiology and hormones, a theme taken up by Myrna Lewis in a later essay on the health status of older women (Lewis 1985). No doubt the definitive case for men as the weaker sex has yet to be established, but women do appear to have a more protective biology that contributes to their longevity. It might also be said that men's psychology has been found to be less protective.

Object relations theory suggests that men are more prone to anomie in terms of some of the dilemmas in the way in which they have resolved the oedipal crisis. In marriage and in work, this vulnerability is often covered over until there is a crisis like divorce or premature and involuntary retirement (McIntosh *et al.* 1997).

Studies of masculine identity persistently suggest that men are more oriented to competition rather than cooperation, to analysis rather than intuition, to conquest rather than submission, to power rather than dependence, to instrumental rather than expressive behaviour, to logical rather than experiential thinking and utilitarianism rather than affection in their relationships (Gradman 1994). Both retirement and role change in late life marriage, however, are seen to threaten the basis of such identity polarisation, particularly if a man is not comfortable with the emergence of the more feminine side of himself.

Developmental social psychologists from Erikson *et al.* (1986) to Levinson *et al.* (1978) have attempted to explore life tasks and successful resolutions across various stages of the lifecourse, Erikson *et al.*, most famously, characterising late life as the resolution of the problem of 'integrity' versus 'despair'. Lifecourse theorists have particularly explored the centrality of work for men and the degree to which the experience of retirement creates a crisis in their adjustment.

Contemporary work on 'successful/productive ageing', particularly that coming out of the work of Paul and Margaret Baltes at the Max Planck Institute in Berlin, also builds on the notion of positive adaptation to the retirement transition, while also recognising that this is an increasingly societal-wide, not merely an individual transition (Baltes & Baltes 1990).

David Gutmann in an original study in the mid-1980s suggested that there was in fact a crossover between men and women in their roles in middle and late life, spurred by the post parental crisis, with women moving from the 'nurturers' to much more 'virile' older persons, while men move in the opposite direction from 'warriors' to 'peace chiefs', setting up an inherent tension in marriages. Both sexes he claimed became more androgynous—the males more affiliative, the females more assertive. Though some dispute the empirical validity of Gutmann's theorising (Thompson 1994), it appears to hold experiential validity in terms of the experience of older couples in marriage. Gutmann's later work has focused on patterns of adjustment of males/females to the crossover phenomenon in late life marriage related to the man's earlier oedipal socialisation in their family of origin.

Others have challenged the degree to which males do in fact become more androgynous in late life suggesting that personality is more fixed and what adjustments do occur are rather overlays on the original orientation (Solomon & Szwabo 1994).

The development of psychotherapy with older men suggests that there is opportunity for growth in later life but that often the opportunity is resolved in the negative for men (and often for women also) leading to depression or passive dependency.

GUIDELINES FOR INTERVENTION WITH OLDER MEN

In many respects intervention approaches in work with older men will demonstrate some of the same characteristics of intervention with the aged in general with an overlay tailored specifically to their gender needs to the degree that these can be identified and differentiated. Finding the right balance between age and gender appropriateness will determine the effectiveness of these interventions.

Literature on intervention with the aged in general suggests that as individuals get older they become more vulnerable to changes in their external environment (Lawton & Nahemow 1973) and less able to personally adapt to those changing externalities, so that interventions need to be increasingly prosthetic and supportive, adapting to changed individual capabilities rather than expecting major change in the older person (Monk 1981; Lawton 1983). Of course the degree of environmental vulnerability or competence relates very much both to actual age (e.g. whether young old/middle old/oldest old) and general health and social status. While an empowerment orientation might be appropriate at a younger age when someone has their full health faculties and social supports, a more protective stance is warranted in the case of people encountering, for instance, severe dementia or homelessness.

The aged are prone to both primary and secondary losses both in terms of physical function and social support (Silverstone & Burack-Weiss 1983) which they must actively adapt to, or accommodate or compensate for. Baltes and Baltes (1990) in fact suggest that successful ageing is all about how effective their 'selective optimisation with compensation' mechanisms are. As people age they experience decrements in the 'mechanics' around which they must 'strategise'.

In relation to the aged in general, and mental health services in particular, a number of barriers to service access have been noted both in the older person themselves, the service providers and the situation of service (Hooyman & Kiyak 1996; Ozanne 1994). In the mental health field both mental health professionals and older adults themselves may discount physical and emotional symptoms as being expected, age-related changes, thus underreporting symptoms and underdiagnosing disorders (Turk *et al.* 1996). When older people do seek treatment they most often do so from a primary care physician. Compared to women, men are less likely to seek treatment for psychological disorders in general (Turk *et al.* 1996). Gomez (1991) suggests this may be because men do not recognise depression and low general wellbeing as signs of emotional disturbances.

What work has been done on effective intervention design with older men (Barusch & Peak 1997) suggests a number of specific guidelines that are responsive to both masculine identity and age characteristics. Such tailored interventions offer men:

- the opportunity to take an instrumental or strategic role;
- to take a focus which is normative and educative rather than primarily therapeutic;
- high information content;
- emphasis on health promoting activities; and
- utilisation of peer contact, support and review as a preferred mode.

From a community health perspective, note must be taken of the importance of social networks to the maintenance of mental and emotional health, although as Adams (1994) has argued, older men's friendship networks have largely been ignored by researchers. Husaini's (1997) findings pointed to the potential benefit to be gained by working to enlarge supportive networks in order to lower depression and enhance social functioning.

As with other groups, intervention to improve access and utilisation by older men will need to occur at individual, group, organisational and institutional levels (Monk 1981), and will require skills in direct practice, organisational change and policy and program development and implementation. It may also require the undertaking of major research and evaluation efforts targeting perceived service gaps.

In the Australian context, the situation of veterans provides an example of a relatively well studied, supported and mainstream population. Research has focused on the needs of older Second World War as well as the younger Vietnam veterans (Gardner *et al.* 1998; Commonwealth Department of Veterans Affairs 1998). From this work, different kinds of intervention strategies appropriate to their differences in age, health status, interests and experiences have been implemented and evaluated (Clinical Evaluation Review Team 1994). Significantly, a number of quite powerful veteran's groups have been active agents in advocating service interventions and in defining the appropriateness of different strategies.

This work on veterans stands in contrast to the relative absence of research focusing on older Aboriginal men, a population at particularly high risk (Swan & Raphael 1996: Harrison 1997). The entire Aboriginal community has not participated in the demographic revolution that has led to the extension of life for the rest of the Australian population. The implications of the Royal Commission into Aboriginal Deaths in Custody (1991) and the Stolen Children Report (National Inquiry 1997) for understanding the condition of older Aboriginal men remain to be properly explicated.

Though the Federal Government has for over a decade now targeted the Aboriginal aged as a particular population at risk (Commonwealth Department of Health, Housing, Local Government and Community Services 1993) there has been little gender differentiation in service development. It is agreed, however, that services do need to be tailored to the particular needs of local communities in doing whatever it takes to improve the quality of life of Aboriginal older people, and that mainstream models of service delivery are probably not appropriate given the very different health profile and life conditions of the majority of the Aboriginal community (Harrison 1996). Proposed service models have tended to push clustered service developments in purpose-built Aboriginal health/resource centres tailored to the particular needs of local communities whether these be in an isolated central Australian town or metropolitan city. Employment of Indigenous health workers in these services as well as Indigenous outreach workers in mainstream health facilities has also been encouraged. Effective interventions are required to actively interlink both Western and traditional medical practices.

In the 1995 report on Aboriginal and Torres Strait Islander mental health (Swan & Raphael 1996), emphasis was placed on the importance of maintaining older people within their family context and addressing men's specific concerns to be involved in the development of health and mental health programs linked to services in other sectors, such as drug and alcohol and forensic programs. Particular emphasis was given, in terms of programming, to building health through sport and physical fitness activities as well as initiating self-help and support programs for trauma, healing and outreach—'men's business'.

REFLECTIONS ON CONTEMPORARY UNDERSTANDINGS OF OLDER MEN

We have noted earlier that there has tended to be an invisibility in relation to research and theorising on older men. Within such limited theoretical perspectives as exist, individual experiences in terms of linear age/stage normative (often) heterosexist perspectives are privileged. Indeed, Australian research appears to lag behind in addressing the needs of older gay males in comparison to the substantial gerontological literature on this topic in the US and elsewhere noted by Turk et al. (1996). A focus on the complexities of understanding the varieties of masculinities that inhere within and construct gender relations awaits explication. In addition, much of the available research has been undertaken on middle-aged and middle-class professional men and appears somewhat normative, dated and negative in its presentation of men's adaptive capacity in late life. Further, such emphasis on middle-aged and middle-class professional men may not necessarily be helpful in understanding the situation and addressing the needs of particular subpopulations of older men such as the homeless or ethnic aged.

In terms of the development of adequate theory, there are interesting precedents when we consider the impact of the women's movement, particularly that of second-wave feminism dating from the early 1970s. At this time, much research and theorising on women's health and emotional wellbeing was conducted either in relation to work done on men, or implications for women were drawn from the available data on men and applied unquestioningly to women. However, since the 1970s this situation has been the subject of critique as researchers and, most importantly, women themselves have worked to erode the status quo of knowledge production and generation. The wealth of studies produced have been instrumental in changing the ways in which all aspects of women's lives have been studied and understood. The importance of this work to considerations of theory development, policy, innovative service provision, and changes in the conditions of many women's lives should not be underestimated.

As we have demonstrated in our mapping of the available literature on older men in relation to social and health provisions, there is a marked absence of older men being studied 'in their own right', as agents and subjects whose interpretations of their own needs have been recognised. Existing objective criteria used to identify their needs, with reference to their biological differences from women, their lifestyle and health habits, their illness behaviour, their health reporting behaviours (Mathers 1994), whilst useful also reveals an important gap in our knowledge base.

DIRECTIONS FOR RESEARCH, POLICY AND SERVICE DEVELOPMENT

In order for practitioners to consider the kinds of interventions or treatment strategies that may be most appropriate for assisting older men who experience problems in their lives, there is a pressing need for an adequate theorisation of the lives and conditions of this age group. Indeed, the lack of knowledge about the experiences of older men during earlier periods in their lives and the impact such lived experiences have on the ways in which older men interpret their present situations and current needs suggests that this is where research must start. In particular, the kind of research that contextualises their experiences as agents and as citizens and is attentive to factors pertaining to gender, class and ethnicity is imperative. Research that focuses on process and participation by older men themselves is essential to the evocation of a critical consciousness among older men, developing and maintaining their capacity as agents. Only from this basis will the possibility for eroding contemporary social constructions of ageing with their oppressive and gender neutral prescriptions be possible. This may be the first of many steps towards policy development and structural change. It may also provide us with the insights we currently lack as to the nature, type and location of services for older men. Such service development has a greater chance of accurately reflecting their interpretation of their own needs at this point in their lives.

The implications of an adequate theorisation of older men as active subjects are many. For example, it may be appropriate, as

Turk *et al.* (1996) have suggested, to integrate feminist perspectives into therapy with older people. Adopting a feminist perspective would enable the service provider to focus on social roles, including the loss of roles such as that of worker or physically healthy person, to recognise gender differences in relation to role, and to demonstrate a sensitivity to the loss of power and status which may accompany the ageing process.

This endeavour reflects, on a practice level, the pro-feminist argument put by May (1998). May advocates the development of a 'progressive male standpoint' from which men can critique their lived experience and the roles they have traditionally adopted. May's contribution is work-in-progress towards the achievement of a 'new vision of what men can become' (May 1998, p. 351). His argument is directed towards reconceptualising male roles, both building on the strengths of these roles and subjecting them to a critique which disturbs the status quo and enables other ways for men to think and to behave, to emerge.

CONCLUSIONS

We have endeavoured to argue in this chapter that older men continue to be somewhat invisible in gerontological and sociological research in Australia, and when they are studied, tend to be predominantly compared to women, rather than studied in their own right, in all their diversity. What theorising has occurred in relation to older men has also tended to be somewhat normative and conservative, based on fairly middle-class populations, and lacking a critical structural analysis. Even political economy theorists (Phillipson 1996; Walker 1980; Guillemard 1993) have not focused particularly on the situation of older men except around the issue of unemployment/retirement. Older men themselves have also not figured as the primary agents of research, their situation tending to have been analysed from without.

In the next twenty years it may be the case that future cohorts of older men will have been influenced by the men's movement, HIV/AIDS, and more sophisticated early gender socialisation and ongoing health education. From this experience it is possible that a different social psychology in late life may emerge with different consequences for the kinds of health and welfare services that become relevant. It may also be that effective health interventions over time will begin to equalise the sex ratio allowing both sexes more chances of intimacy and support in late life. The future might also see older men initiate and participate in work to understand the conditions of their own lives, enabling the emergence of radically different theorisations and actions to meet their own challenges and interpretations of need.

The field of men's health in late life is a growing and at times controversial one (Rubinstein 1996). Of necessity, this chapter has been selective in its coverage, mapping rather than detailing specific points of importance. While increased understanding of the contributions of biology, social psychology, environment, and health behaviour may ensure interventions are effective, we also argue that the prevailing lines of inquiry into older men's health require critique. A perspective that moves beyond comparative methodologies and enables older men themselves to contribute actively to the development of theory and practice is imperative.

14 | The changing role of Indigenous men in community and family life: A conversation between *Graham Atkinson*[1] *and Bob Pease*

Maybe a place to start would be for you to give some background about yourself and the kind of work that you do.

I was born in Echuca, Victoria, and just had my 52nd birthday in January this year. I am a member of the Victorian Koori or Indigenous community and also native title holder and clan member of the Yorta Yorta and Dja Dja Wurrung clans. Late last year the Yorta Yorta appealed against the Federal Court's determination at the end of 1998 that declined to recognise our native title claim for the Barmah Forest and remaining crown land on our traditional tribal land that encompassed a large part of the south-eastern Loddon Mallee, southern Riverina, Goulburn Valley and north-eastern Victoria regions.[2] Central to the Yorta Yorta claim area are the Murray, Campaspe and Edwards river systems. On both my mother's and father's side, I am a descendant of Kitty Atkinson/Cooper[3] who the Federal Court recognised as one the two chief ancestors of the claim. My early ancestors were river and forest people.

Both my mother and father were ambi-lineal in that they had ancestral roots not only with the Yorta Yorta but also with the Djara or Loddon Tribe people that Clark subsumed under the language group, Dja Dja Wurrung.[4] This name has become synonymous with the Djara people who occupied a large area encompassing the Central Highlands and surrounding escarpments of the Loddon region. Our traditional tribal territories stretch from Mt Macedon, across to Daylesford, arching around Maryborough, Charlton, Burchip, across to Boort then Pyramid Hill before returning south and passing just east of Bendigo back towards Mt Macedon. Key land marks of the Dja Dja Wurrung were not only the central highlands and rocky escarpments but also the valleys and water ways such as the Campaspe, Loddon and Avoca river systems. My maternal great grandfather, Henry Harmony Nelson, was born at Majorca, just near Maryborough during the Great Gold Rush in 1851. He spent a short time with Edward Stone Parker[5] at Franklinford Aboriginal Mission near Mt Franklin before its closure and its remaining occupants moved to Correnderk Aboriginal Station near Healsville in the early 1860s. My paternal great grandmother, Caroline Malcom-Morgan, was born in Dja Dja Wurrung country around the same time as my great grandfather. The Dja Dja Wurrung were one of the five Kulin nations who frequently met in the site that is now Melbourne prior to and after occupation to discuss tribal business and perform ceremonies. These lasted many days before each nation, the Wurundjeri, Benerong, Tungerong, Wutherong and Dja Dja Wurrung then dispersed to their own country.

With such a rich history as this, it is no wonder that I have devoted most of my adult life to Aboriginal affairs. I would say though that my involvement in Aboriginal affairs started from when I was born. Growing up during my childhood and teenage years in Echuca always meant coming face to face with overt and covert racism, marginalisation and exclusion. These were my constant companions and informal day-to-day experiences as a Koori person growing up in a non-Koori society.

Becoming actively involved in Koori affairs began in the early 1970s when I commenced studies in social work at Melbourne University. During the university holidays, I got involved with the local Koori community in the metropolitan area.

When I started my course at Melbourne University, studying community development, group structures and community organisation, I developed a framework that helped me work with the Koori community. My involvement has continued throughout the last 25 years or more. After I graduated from Melbourne University in 1977 the Victorian Regional Office of the Department of Aboriginal Affairs appointed me to the position of Community Advisor for the Melbourne metropolitan region. My responsibility included liaising with the newly established Aboriginal peak organisations such as the Victorian Aboriginal Medical Service, Victorian Aboriginal Legal Service, Victorian Aborigines Advancement League, Victorian Aboriginal Child Care Agency[6] and Victorian Aboriginal Cooperative. I left the Department of Aboriginal Affairs in 1978 after being appointed by the Victorian Aboriginal Child Care Agency to its Senior Social Worker position. I eventually became Program Manager of VACCA before the recently formed Aboriginal Development Commission appointed me as Regional Director for its Victoria and Tasmania Regional Office based in Melbourne in 1981, which I left in 1986 to set up my own private consulting business. So for the last fourteen years I have been managing and operating my business, which in 1994 became Yuruga Enterprises Pty Ltd, an Indigenous owned and controlled consulting and training firm. I completed my Bachelor of Arts from Melbourne University in 1981 and my Masters in Business Administration (MBA) at RMIT in 1994.

Can you say something about what specific projects you've recently been involved in?

My company, Yuruga, has recently undertaken a joint evaluation with the University of Melbourne's School of Social Work of the Aboriginal Family Preservation Pilot Program for the Department of Human Services' Care and Protection Branch. The Department is piloting the program in the Loddon-Mallee, Hume and Central Morwell regions. The evaluation team is just nearing the closing stages of the two-year study. Significantly, this project has exposed the team to a range of issues concerning Aboriginal child safety and wellbeing, out of home placements or extended care, and a wide range of structural and social problems that impact on the limited resources of the preservation services such as domestic family violence, alcohol and substance abuse, unemployment, accommodation shortages, disconnected and alienated youth, homelessness, mental health and school truancy. One area that has been highlighted by service workers is the impact of dominant society on the role of Aboriginal men and the underlying issues of their sense of powerlessness.

There is a view that Indigenous men's roles were affected more by white invasion and colonisation than Indigenous women's roles. Can you say something about that?

A strong theme that emerges from Koori history and the impact of colonisation is the unequal status of Aboriginal men and women. In terms of the influence that Aboriginal women have asserted, particularly in Aboriginal organisations, it has historically been more dominant than Aboriginal men. I think this is because women have been able to use their 'femininity' and 'womanly drive and ingenuity' to their advantage to empower themselves to achieve things for their families and local community. The irony here is that where Aboriginal men have resorted to using their masculinity, apart from on the sporting field, to compete equally with main-stream Australia, they were often viewed as a threat by their non-Aboriginal male counterparts. My father, who was a shearer in his early adult life, often lamented that Aboriginal men were quickly reminded of their place at the bottom of the pecking order. In contrast I think that non-Aboriginal society, particularly male society, gave Aboriginal women more recognition for their achievements and contribution than for Aboriginal men. That is, the recognition and tacit support that non-Aboriginal society selectively bestowed on Aboriginal women, particularly in the urban or semi-urban context, elevated many of them to certain levels of influence and power within their own communities.

My own family experience is a good example here. My mother, because of her drive and her 'take no crap' attitude to life, managed to gain the respect and recognition from the wider community in Echuca where we lived and in the Goulburn Valley area where she spent her early adult years. Never shy to assert her rights in whatever company she found herself in, or task she had to undertake, she always managed to achieve things for her family, whether it be securing a cooking position at the local hospital, mixing socially with all walks of life or raising her seven children on a meagre income. She battled and struggled day and night to ensure her family's wellbeing was taken care of. In my early days of living in Echuca there were other Aboriginal women who attained the same recognition but I do not have the same memories of Aboriginal men in the town achieving the same results. There were obviously Aboriginal men of character who did command respect, but they seemed disproportionately less than Aboriginal women. Most Aboriginal men in those days were conveniently marginalised to the 'out of sight out of mind' category.

The answers to this are embedded in our history. We know that Aboriginal women and men were exploited economically, socially and in the case of women, sexually, particularly when they were forced from the missions to provide domestic labour for nearby pastoral stations. Yet Koori men, even though their labour contributed to the local pastoral industry, often worked on isolated properties many miles from local townships. The property owners kept Aboriginal workers away from their homesteads and families by assigning them tasks in isolated sections of the farm. The concept of mateship and egalitarianism didn't necessarily extend to Aboriginal males, it mainly referred to white men. The social controls that were applied to Aboriginal farm labourers, particularly in their limited opportunities for relations with non-Koori women, suggest that white property owners perceived Aboriginal men as a threat, perhaps sexually. This gave rise to property owners and other farm workers subordinating and denigrating the status of Aboriginal men. I would call the process a systematic subordination and put-down of the Koori man's role and status in the community.

The life expectancy of Indigenous men in Australia is eighteen years below that of non-Indigenous men. Can you say something about what you see as the major forces contributing to Indigenous men's ill-health?

When you examine how Aboriginal men were marginalised immediately after European occupation, it had a destructive impact on men, not only socially but physically and psychologically. It must have been soul destroying to be constantly reminded that you were unequal, inferior and not worthy. Strong feelings of inferiority in relation to non-Aboriginal male society led to the self-perception they were no longer a key player in their family and community. The resulting sense of inferiority was further reinforced by their status of unskilled or a cheap labour source. For example, what could a third grade mission education offer a young Aboriginal man aspiring to seek work in the mainstream labour market? The mission system entrenched the barriers to equal employment and opportunity because most if not all Aboriginal men up until the mid-twentieth century were only able to find unskilled or labouring work. For example, my father followed the same pattern as his father and grandfather. All were educated to grade three level on the Cummeragunja Mission, established in the 1870s just across the river from Barmah. Young thirteen- and fourteen-year-old boys and girls were indentured to work on the Moira Station, one of the largest pastoral runs in the area. My grandfather, Henry Atkinson, became a shepherd and boundary rider. Riding out for miles to patch up fences and herding sheep were tasks that occupied his time for weeks and even months on end before he would be called back to the homestead. As with many Aboriginal men who worked at Moira Station, he learned shearing. When my father arrived at Moira Station he learned to shear from his father. The *Aborigines Protection Act of 1869 and 1886* enshrined the systematic policy and practice of indenturing young boys and girls on local stations where they often worked for rations rather than wages. Perhaps the only positive thing that the local pastoral properties saw in Aboriginal men was that they were good at working on the surrounding farms.

What were the main consequences of these living conditions?

The isolation, coupled with the ethos of the hard-working shearer, led to drinking to fill in the time in the evenings and at weekends. Away for long periods, they would not see their families for weeks, sometimes months. I think in that particular industry in earlier days, the notion of mateship often manifested itself in negative ways. Alcohol became not only a tool to fill the idle hours or deaden the pain of homesickness, it was used to prove one's manhood. Like the influence of earlier introduced diseases that Aboriginal people were not immune from, Anglo-European behaviours like the above sooner or later impacted on Aboriginal men's lifestyles. My father became an alcoholic because of his experiences, which in turn affected his physical and mental health. This in turn affected his relationship with my mother. Relationships in other families reflected similar behaviours and patterns.

Can you say something more about the impact on those relationships?

To mask their low self-esteem, alienated Aboriginal men like my father resorted to heavy drinking bouts that invariably led to conflict and rows with their female partners. This volatile situation often erupted in family violence, followed the next day by guilt, remorse and self-pity. With little sense of self-worth and raging inferiority complexes, men's problems were rarely resolved, they often worsened. Aboriginal wives and partners perhaps gained some respite or false sense of security when their husbands returned to the shearing shed or went looking for work in nearby townships. I often think of the Aboriginal women and families caught in this predicament wishfully thinking that their partners would return cured men when the shearing season or work finished. But the problems rarely resolved themselves.

When the station work tapered off Aboriginal men struggled to find permanent work in the townships, except for unskilled or labouring jobs. So when we consider the accumulated effect of colonisation, marginalisation, subordination and the impact of the dominant culture on Koori men, the present status of Koori men is all too obvious.

The present dysfunctional family behaviours that our evaluation of the Aboriginal Family Preservation Program has found can be linked to the pressures and traumas that Aboriginal people and their forebears have endured due to the impact of European occupation and dominant non-Aboriginal culture. Many of the negative self-destructive behaviours learned by families to cope with their traumatic circumstances are more often than not cyclical and intergenerational. Families that harbour the propensity for unstable relationships or fragmented relationships usually have histories of children being removed, disengagement, alienation, coupled with alcohol and substance abuse. Similar patterns of behaviour are transferred to the next family offspring.

Have there been any programs developed specifically to work with men in relation to these issues?

The sort of services introduced by State and Federal Governments have tended to be generic programs. For instance, alcohol and drug services that have been established work with people who have alcohol and substance abuse problems. But staff work with both women and men, not necessarily one or the other. Exceptions to this though are the network of women's refuges and some of the detoxification and drying out centres that are male or female specific.

While there have been specific services established in the specialised areas such as alcohol and drug support, my anecdotal information is that they have had limited success. One problem is that these programs are not set up properly in the first place. The common issues apply—limited resourcing and funding and engagement of untrained or unskilled staff. Rigorous planning for these services is often absent which means they are all too frequently set up in an ad hoc way, often as a reaction to the problem. At the human resource level, the services often employ people at the service delivery level who are not experienced or trained in dealing with these complex problems. This approach would also apply to setting up a men's specific service. Though I am aware of attempts in various areas of Victoria to establish men's groups, they have never had the success of other Koori services such as health, housing, legal, education and social support. A men's camp was held in 1999 at the Warakoo Station, 80 kilometres from Wentworth. This is a Victorian program that was funded by the Aboriginal and Torres Strait Islander Commission (ATSIC) to deal with young offenders.

What was the purpose of that gathering?

The aim of the men's camp was to bring people together to encourage men to start talking about some of their underlying problems of alcoholism, substance abuse, family violence, men's health issues, broader health issues, their role in the community and to provide a support base for each other. The idea of the camp is a positive one, but it is the follow-up and actions that need to be implemented that counts in the end. Some meetings achieve results but all too frequently many good ideas and intentions either get left at the meeting or are never effectively followed up.

Implicit in the notion of Koori men's groups seems to be a feeling of Aboriginal men who have historically been subordinated, seeking to empower themselves to raise their status in the community. Also for them to have more positive influence in their families, communities and Koori organisation network on how the services are managed and organised.

Have women been supportive and encouraging of these developments among Koori men?

Aboriginal women's support for Aboriginal men's groups appears to have been mixed. I would suggest that Aboriginal women who have had positive and constructive experiences with their male counterparts are supportive and have tried to establish an equal relationship with men. However, I would also suggest that women who have had negative or destructive experiences in their relationships with Koori males seem to take a more defensive position on how they relate to Koori men. This is understandable, particularly from women who have been victims of not just physically but also emotionally violent relationships. Many still carry a lot of scars and baggage with them, which colours their perception of Koori men and largely determines the extent to which they interact with or avoid men. My own experience in working with women who have been victims is that the defences are not too far away. They are certainly there if they feel threatened by Koori males.

How is the issue of men's violence against women within Indigenous communities understood? Is it seen predominantly as a consequence of colonisation?

There are different schools of thought on the origins of domestic violence in the Aboriginal community. In our community it is more referred to as family violence. This gives the connotation that violence affects the whole family. It doesn't just confine itself to the parents in a family situation. It invariably involves the immediate family and the extended family. Judy Atkinson has written a lot on the origins of family violence.[7] She relates it to the impact of colonisation and the effect that had on Aboriginal men. Her view is that family violence before white invasion or occupation was unknown in the Aboriginal community. Colonisation involved the oppression of Aboriginal communities and disempowerment[8] of Aboriginal men. Violence within the family emerged as a reaction to the impact of an alien dominant culture.

In the white community, in the last ten years, one of the ways of addressing men's violence has been to develop counselling and education groups for perpetrators. What sort of developments have occurred in Koori communities?

In Koori children's and family services, staff will deal with the victims, the women and the children. They won't necessarily deal with the perpetrator. In fact they shield their clients from any contact with the male perpetrator. For example, when the mother and kids are accommodated in a safe house or a refuge, their privacy, confidentiality and security is guarded closely. No men in the community, even myself, know where these places are. However, some staff will interact with other service providers, perhaps other members of the perpetrator's family, elders or other male figures in the community, to talk to the perpetrator. Because this is a loose structure, follow-up work is often done informally and consequently suffers the risk of no follow through.

At this stage there do not appear to be any formal linkages between the women who are involved in domestic violence services and the men's group movement. There is an issue here of direct or third party contacts. Usually people involved in those services will safeguard the interests of women. However, they will use other contacts, often Koori men's contacts, to look after the interests of the male partner or the perpetrator.

I come from a family where family violence was a big issue in my early childhood and early teenage years. When I reflect on how my family dealt with it in those days, it was quite interesting. Because it affected both our immediate and extended family the women and girls in the family would shield or support my mother from our father's violent behaviour. It was an unspoken expectation that the men and my brothers would try to counsel my father. Even his friends, his cousins, relatives and people like that would take him aside and talk to him and say that behaviour that disrupted the family wasn't on.

Often someone would emerge as the mediator. The eldest daughter in the family would try to mediate between both my parents. She would tell my father off, have stern words with him. However, in hindsight, when I assess whether that was a good structure for dealing with family violence, I would have to conclude that it wasn't effective. It was an informal structure. If mum called the authorities such as the police when things got out of hand they were reluctant to intervene, particularly when they could see other informal networks trying to deal with the problem. I arrive at this conclusion because my parents' relationship became very violent in the end and eventually broke down. It is tempting to drift back to the idyllic times when Aboriginal people themselves or communities used traditional practices to resolve these complex issues. Unfortunately, many traditional or cultural practices here in Victoria suffered from colonisation, leaving a gap for dealing with complex problems like human relationships. A void exists today that has to be filled to address these problems but in culturally appropriate ways.

What would a culturally appropriate way of addressing the problem look like in your view?

The safety of the mother and her human rights are paramount. Perhaps we need to move from insular local approaches to more general or global remedies such as the assertion of Aboriginal people's human rights. Like all groups and societies, Aboriginal people are entitled to the preservation of their human rights. So protection and safety is paramount in that context. An effective culturally appropriate structure is a service delivery system that employs and trains skilled Aboriginal workers or non-Aboriginal workers who use a bi-cultural focus that encompasses both Indigenous and non-Indigenous cultures. The term bi-cultural means the opposite to mono-cultural perspective on practice issues. For example, the evaluation team of the Aboriginal Family Preservation Program mentioned earlier, found that its staff who operated from a bi-cultural perspective proved to be one of its key strengths. It helped them to more effectively negotiate both culturally-based systems.

Can you talk a bit more about men's business and women's business? The sense that I have is that it is more than just a separation of gender-specific functions and a code of conduct for men and women.

We know that traditionally Aboriginal men were the hunters and women were the gatherers. While this provided a useful comparison of the different roles, it goes much deeper than that. On a personal level I know of many Koori men who are reluctant to talk about their personal issues with a woman, particularly a Koori woman. And I know it's the same for Koori women. They prefer to discuss these things with their own gender. For instance, when I worked for VACCA in the late 1970s, when I counselled women or young girls, I always intuitively sensed a barrier when we talked about sensitive matters.

There is an unwritten code for dealing with men's and women's business. I know from my own cultural experience most Aboriginal people 'know' the difference. It's not written down on paper. It is knowledge gained through one's socialisation. Our parents and elders taught us that gender differences have to be respected and acknowledged. I can recall observing the differences, particularly in various social contexts. For example, when Koori women socialise they behave differently in a group and the same applies to Koori men. In mixed company with non-Aboriginal people their behaviour is different again, perhaps not as informal or free spirited as when they are with their own.

You mentioned before that the men's gathering was a beginning attempt for men to acknowledge that they had a responsibility to address these issues. Can you say a bit more about that?

I think this was one of the key purposes but I am concerned about the follow-up process to put the words into actions. Another issue that is often overlooked is the power relations between men and women. There are exceptions to this. For instance, some Koori men to whom I have spoken feel they have equal relationships with Koori or non-Koori women. But others feel they have a less dominant role or less equal role to Koori and non-Koori women. I think the underlying agenda in the former is about equal partnerships but in the latter it's about gaining more control of family and community structures. Although it has not been articulated in this way I think power and control are common issues that my community still needs to sort out.

It sounds very similar to the men's movement in the non-Indigenous community. Do you see any parallels there?

What I've experienced in Aboriginal affairs is the 'lag effect' in relation to broader trends. In other words the trends when they influence the Koori community trigger a delayed reaction. For example, when mainstream community goes down a certain path, it may be three, four or five years later when the Koori community arrives at the same turning point. The Koori community will then in some cases replicate, but in a more culturally appropriate way, those same directions and themes. This has emerged particularly in child protection. In the early days when VACCA began, I constantly heard both Aboriginal and non-Aboriginal activists asserting that traditional remedies would solve the problem of child abuse in the Koori community. But these were often esoteric remedies based more on idealistic notions than actual practice. Yet some Aboriginal people now who work at the coal face of child protection seem to have lost faith or confidence in earlier family practices and sometimes see 'removing the child' as the only option when all else has failed. It is often because the structures that are assumed to be there aren't there. Of course it is a measure of last resort, but if your priority is the child's safety and wellbeing, sometimes that is the only option workers have got. However, the possibility of removal in early 1980s was taboo, in some cases it wasn't the 'politically correct' thing to even contemplate. You couldn't even mention that option. In the area of alcohol and substance abuse and family preservation there are some parallels. What I have found with the evaluation is the gradual convergence between mainstream and Koori practices. For instance, at the pinnacle of family preservation practice is the child's safety, which is clearly now a human rights issue. Regardless of what culture people come from, everyone's entitled to a safe environment.

Have there been any developments where Indigenous men and Indigenous women have worked together on some of these issues?

I think there are instances on the periphery of service structures where women and men are recognising that more effective measures need to be taken to address the problems of family violence, alcohol and substance abuse, and child physical and sexual abuse in our communities. But a more radical shift is required at the decision-making and power centres of services, rather than a chipping away at the edges of those problems. Ironically, in the general community development area some women and men are forging relationships and working more closely together to establish better services.

There still are walls of silence and secrecy on some of these issues that workers need to penetrate, and it's not an easy job. Because of the hurt and pain associated with these issues it is also difficult shifting the spotlight onto those areas.

There seem to have been some very successful projects where Indigenous women and non-Indigenous women have worked together. Do you think that there are possibilities for Indigenous men and non-Indigenous men to work cooperatively on some of these issues?

There are several indirect examples that we could explore. Sport, for example, is one social context where Aboriginal and non-Aboriginal men interact positively. Perhaps the common purpose and common interest that binds both groups overcomes the racial or cultural divide. Another area that falls outside the human services field is music. Once again the common interest or universal language of music brings both groups together. I think also that in the academic or education field, where a meeting of the minds on common issues often takes place, this helps to build bridges as well. Another area is the native title debate. A lot of cross-cultural interaction is happening on this issue at the moment with key bodies such as Defenders of Native Title taking up the cause of Aboriginal people. Because the Aboriginal Family Preservation Program is at an important stage of its development, it has the potential to forge important cross-cultural and service linkages for both women and men and for Aboriginal and non-Aboriginal relationships. Perhaps this has come about through the hands-on experience that staff have gained in the last three years that they've been operating. Through a process of trial and error, they've been able to refine and develop their practice.

Is that a possible model that could be applied to other areas?

It can be. Mainly because the workers in the three pilot services appear to have gone through a learning process themselves. The evaluation team has found that staff have been rigorously discerning in their analysis of mainstream and culturally appropriate practice. It is as if they have assessed both mainstream culture and available services and rather than lock themselves in one particular paradigm, which emotionally says that it is either this or that, they've been able to blend what is appropriate from each model. They have also been adept at deciding when it is appropriate to refer their clients to mainstream services, the precursor being those services that are culturally sensitive. So as well as being culturally appropriate, staff must also have cross-cultural skills.

To bring this conversation to a close, can you say what white male workers can do to be more supportive of Indigenous men's issues?

They need to recognise the systematic practice of exclusion and disempowerment that impacted on Aboriginal men that enabled the dominant culture to subordinate their family role and community status. As I said earlier, Aboriginal men not only had unequal relationships with dominant mainstream culture but also with Aboriginal women, particularly those who forged dominant roles in family and community affairs. They also need to examine some of the assumptions that underpin both the mainstream and Koori service structure. Misunderstandings and barriers between mainstream and Aboriginal service workers often rest on mis-interpretations of negative behaviours such as family violence, child safety issues, alcohol and substance abuse as the norm in Koori culture. White workers also need to be sensitive to the separate areas of men's and women's business in the Koori community. And they need to recognise that change occurs at a different pace to mainstream policies and programs. Finally, they have to recognise that Indigenous rights are inseparable from human rights. So effective services must take into account Indigenous men's history and present needs and also develop partnerships with Aboriginal women's services and wider support services.

15 Rethinking sex and gender in work with gay identified men

Richard Roberts

'Working with men' invites human services practitioners to understand and to deconstruct the meaning of gender, its politics and its practices. 'Working with gay identified men'[1] invites us to understand the influence of sexual orientation and its relationship to gender. As conceptual maps of particular types of behaviour, gender and sexual orientation[2] stand side by side influencing each other. Hence in any writing about human services practices, both should be considered.

Until challenged by various waves of feminism, 'being male' was considered important, desirable and to be strived for (even, or especially, by some women). To bolster a patriarchal system of power relationships, male gender traits and roles were constructed as superior (Kimmel 1994), and language genderised so that it defaulted to the masculine form. Enjoying a similar superiority was the sexual orientation of 'heterosexual'. Its opposite, 'homosexual', was viewed not so much as inferior (as some might view female gender traits and roles), but rather subversive, deviant, abnormal and immoral (see, for example, Thompson 1985; Greenberg 1988; Garnets & Kimmel 1993). The challenge of working within a heterosexual hegemony is not only to raise the consciousness of others to the human rights issues as they apply to all parts of the community, but to lift the discourse from illegal, immoral and abnormal paradigms into legal, amoral and normal ones. Any consideration of practices for working with gay identified men must deal with a social context that remains conservative of heterosexist dynamics and where discourses of 'equal but different' are still emerging. This is despite contemporary legislative and human rights reforms that recognise gay men and our rights.[3]

This chapter will be divided into three main parts. In the first section I will outline important themes that form part of the social context of working with gay identified men. The second section will deal with specific challenges for the practitioner, including the need for practitioner self-awareness and the dangers of confusing gender and sexual orientation. In the third section, I will deal with common problems faced by gay men, including 'coming out', achieving intimacy, and dealing with homophobia.

A BACKDROP TO INTERPERSONAL HELPING

At least in the rhetoric of human service professions, attempts have been made to acknowledge the importance of the social context in which individual concerns are located (for example, Roberts 1990). Through this acknowledgment, phenomena can be viewed as socially constructed, relative and permeable. A failure to recognise this reinforces individual pathology so that problems and issues are seen to be carried by the individual, are viewed as more or less his[4] fault, and solutions to these problems and issues are seen to come from within. This essentialist position ignores cultural and sub-cultural relativities and ignores the influence of meaning and context on problem definition and solutions. While the delineation of individual differences will help to determine the different ways individual gay men react to and influence their social environments, it is important for the practitioner to understand some general features that permeate many individual personal concerns to some degree or another.

In defining a particular group by an attribute such as 'gay identity' there is always the danger that this marker will be interpreted as construing those people within it as 'different' just because of their sexual orientation. To some extent this is so. However, in order for the practitioner to be effective at an individual level, it is important that each man is recognised as having a potentially wide range of other characteristics pertaining, for example, to his social class, socioeconomic status, education, life interests and other proclivities (Roberts 2000). Furthermore, sexual orientation is more properly described as 'sexualities' to give credence to the multifarious forms of sexual expression and behaviour resulting from a gay identity. In the counselling context the delineation of the specific aspects of the client's location in terms of his sexual orientation as well as the other trajectories of his life is an important and essential precursor to a viable social assessment.

Having recognised the influence of these differences (both individual and contextual), it is a next step to observe how a particular sexual identity has been shaped. In working with this client group it can be easy to assume (at least covertly) that because of their sexual identity, all gay men will be relatively similar in their world views and in their behaviours. Such a position invariably will lead to ill-conceived assumptions and sweeping generalisations. This unitary view helps form the myths about, for example, gay men's predatory sexual behaviours, high disposable incomes, 'unstable' intimate relationships and so on. Unquestioned, these assumptions can camouflage the exact type of request being made by the client, the client's definition of his situation that leads to his seeking help, and the particular attributes, resources and deficits that will influence the client in working towards a solution.

This diversity in the social fabric has long been recognised at the sociological level (Thompson 1985; Garnets & Kimmel 1993). However, in engaging in any form of interpersonal work with gay men it is important for the practitioner to facilitate his or her client to enunciate how he locates himself and his individual differences within a social fabric. It is only when these differences can be acknowledged that their influence on gay identity issues can be fully appreciated as well as the way in which the client's 'gay sexuality' can be appreciated as just one set of variables nestled in alongside many others.

Having acknowledged this richness and diversity in the social fabric and acknowledged that fact for a group defined as gay identified men, it is very important that the meaning of that social context for each client is explicated. How much is a person's life structured around their sexual identity, for example? For some gay men their identity as gay is worked out very closely with the friendships and relationships they form, where they live, where they socialise, where (or if) they vacation and so on. This is epitomised in the emergence of the gay ghetto or more broadly in a 'gay community' surpassing geographic boundaries. For other gay men, however, their gay identity is only very loosely connected with other parts of their lives. For these men, they might remain close to their heterosexual families of origin, their heterosexual friendship networks, or gay couples might blend into a suburban heterosexual family lifestyle. 'Coming out' for these men may be construed as far less important, and some may choose not to identify as 'gay', although they remain sexually attracted to other men.

A second defining contextual variable, operating alongside the individual meaning attributed to a client's situation and context, is the pervasiveness of homophobia (Cox 1990; Schembri 1992; Mason & Tomsen 1997; Cox 1994; Lesbian and Gay Community Action of South Australia 1994; NSW Police Service 1995). This recognition needs to acknowledge the effects not only of individual forms of homophobia, such as prejudice or violence directed against gay identified men, but also the structural inequalities that have been constructed based on belief systems that posit gay identity and/or behaviour as immoral, illegal and/or socially and sexually deviant. Such an acknowledgment, even within contemporary contexts of revision, recognises the strong influences upon client and practitioner alike, and has an effect on the behaviour of both. Despite liberally constructed codes of ethics (see, for example, AASW Code of Ethics 1999) many human service practitioners remain homophobic (Faria 1997; Berkman & Zinberg 1997; Appleby & Anastas 1998), and despite highly visible advocacy in other human rights arenas, gay issues are still often omitted from mainstream 'rights' agendas.

CHALLENGES FOR THE PRACTITIONER

While practitioner self-awareness is a vital component of effective interpersonal helping with any client or client group, there are added challenges in working with gay men. Like sexism and racism, homophobia has some effect on us all (Bluemfeld 1992), even for self-aware and gay identified gay clients and practitioners. Given an effective socialisation into heterosexist values, it is often difficult to appreciate how inequality can be perceived and the effects it has. Covert homophobia can affect the practitioner by his or her ignorance of issues relevant to gay men particularly as these issues are diversified within this sub-culture. This type of homophobia can be reflected in the practitioner's inability to move beyond the orthodox.

Another challenge for the practitioner is to be able to under-stand the difference between sexual orientation and sexual identity, as well as the ways in which these conceptual tools link to each other. Gender refers to an identification of behaviours that signify whether one is male or female. Masculine gender traits are those traits that describe 'male like' behaviours. These behaviours are often associated with particular gender roles and both traits and roles together serve to describe and prescribe how men and women will or should behave in relation to their 'maleness' and 'female-ness'. While gender ascriptions vary from culture to culture, and often from sub-culture to sub-culture, they serve to reinforce differential power relations between genders. Hence the cost of non-conformity is usually very high, and the process of changing these norms long and difficult. This is very much in evidence in the process of creating greater equality between women and men.

On the other hand, sexual orientation refers to an individual person's preference to engage in sexual behaviour with another person, regardless of that person's gender. Sexual orientation is usually constructed as a continuum between primarily homosexual through to primarily heterosexual with varying degrees of bisex-uality in between (see, for example, the Kinsey scale, in Masters, Johnson & Kolodny 1988). While many agree that the prevalence of and potential for bisexual behaviour is high, in a heterosexist society, only those attributes and behaviours that are seen as heterosexual are valued, so that other bisexual and homosexual behaviours are at best marginalised and at worst stigmatised and punished.

The most common source of confusion between sexual orien-tation and gender occurs where effeminate gender traits are interpreted as gay identity. Such a confusion arises when mascu-line gender traits are uncritically linked to heterosexuality. By default, non-masculine gender traits must be linked with non-heterosexuality. This confusion is well documented in the discrim-ination literature, where non-masculine men are more likely to be bullied or called pejorative names in public because their behaviour is assumed to represent homosexuality (see, for example, Roberts 1995; 1996). On the other hand, many gay men with masculine gender traits may 'pass' as heterosexual, unless specific inquiry is made by the practitioner, or these men choose to 'come out'.

In passing, it should be noted that sexual orientation can be confused with cross-dressing (transvestism) and with trans-genderism. In reality, a proportion of both gay and straight men cross-dress from time to time, either occasionally or regularly. Those who are trans-gender, with or without reassignment, may identify as 'gay' *or* 'straight'. On each axis, an assessment needs to be made, rather than assuming that *any* 'atypical' behaviour is indicative of some form of homosexuality.

Sexual orientation and gender differentiation can also be illustrated by reference to gendered behaviours within particular gay sub-cultures where the term 'straight-acting' is used to refer to masculine (or perhaps even 'macho') gender characteristics. Within these particular sub-cultures it seems that masculine gender traits are prised above non-masculine ones, and forms of 'hyper-masculinity' that can be observed in some contemporary Western gay sub-cultures and represented by highly muscularised, defined, and lean bodies, held high on the list of desirable personal attributes. Explanations for this type of behaviour may centre on the need to compensate for the anorexic body image associated with HIV infection, or the need to project images of strength in the face of personal violence and harassment. On the other hand, it may be a reaction to the common association of being gay with effeminate mannerisms—a position that clearly denigrates feminine gender traits.

The point for the practitioner to appreciate is that sexual orientation can never be assumed. It can be established only by inquiry, or by a person 'coming out'. Reliance on gender characteristics that are visible is highly unreliable as an indicator of sexual orientation.

The remainder of this chapter will be devoted to a discussion of common issues brought by gay men to counselling and common approaches to dealing with these problems.

'COMING OUT'

As already noted above, sexual orientation can only be established by inquiry or the volunteering of this information by the client. Observation (particularly of gender traits) in the absence of other corroboration may give an inconclusive or inaccurate impression. Furthermore, there are sub-groups of men who engage in sexual behaviours with other men but who do not identify as gay. 'Situational homosexuality' in same-sex institutions and some 'men who have sex with other men' often in public and semi-public male spaces, are examples. The problems faced by non-gay identifying men who have sex with other men[5] often centre on their juggling of their homosexual or bisexual behaviours within the expectations of, or their identity with, heterosexuality. This may involve the challenges of 'staying in the closet' and constructing a 'double life'. While the needs and problems of non-gay identified men who have sex with men should not be marginalised, the issues remain somewhat different and will not be dealt with further here.

For the gay identified man, a central challenge is 'coming out' (Minton & McDonald 1985). Such a phenomenon has no equivalent for the straight man in a heterosexist society, because the expectation is that all men are or should be heterosexual. Heterosexual status is unremarkable and assumed. In addition, rather than being a one-off event, 'coming out' usually involves a life-long process with many 'coming outs' throughout the lifecycle and in different social contexts. It may be extensive or highly selective. The stages of the 'coming out' process have been researched and documented (Minton & McDonald 1985; Coleman 1985; Cass 1979) and I do not propose to repeat this material here. From a therapeutic viewpoint, 'coming out' usually needs to be planned and strategic and its consequences anticipated and planned for. Unlike their heterosexual counterparts, there are few well-established rites of passage for gay men, resulting in the need to individually construct 'coming out' events to suit the individual person's circumstances and wishes.

From a practice perspective, there are two central issues to be dealt with. The first centres on the consequences of 'coming out' for the individual client. The second issue centres on the reactions of others to the client's 'coming out' and how the client is able to deal with and reach some resolution to the reactions of significant others (Mallon 1994). It must be acknowledged that the majority of people who 'come out' are able to do so without the need for professional assistance. However, for those who seek help, it is important that the practitioner is able to help the client to become more insightful into the process of 'coming out' as an individual matter, but also to be aware of that personal process in relation to the reactions of significant others. The reactions of others can cover a wide domain from total acceptance to total rejection sometimes associated with physical and emotional violence.

Rather than constructing the process as universal, the practitioner must attempt to individualise each client's particular situation (Garnets & Kimmel 1993). For the young man, still in adolescence, the additional trauma of having to deal with a sexual confusion that is subject to explicit societal approbation can often result in a 'delayed adolescence' (Johnson 1996) on the one hand, or an inability to cope with the demands of everyday life, including schooling (Roberts 1996), on the other. There is evidence that failure to successfully resolve this challenge is one factor in the high rate of youth suicide especially in rural areas (Hershberger *et al.* 1997; Anderson 1998). However tragic, this situation may be no more traumatic than the situation of a middle-aged man, coming to terms with his sexual identity and having to 'come out' to his wife and children, and then set about re-establishing his life situation in the face of his newly acknowledged homosexuality. Both these situations involve different dynamics, and while both involve 'coming out', the coping capacities, access to resources, and the ability to deal with a potentially hostile environment may well be very different. While it can be argued that there is much to be gained from 'coming out', at both a personal and political level, and the alternative of dealing with the politics and personal constraints of the closet are just as challenging (Sedgwick 1990), nevertheless, from a clinical viewpoint, the decision to 'come out' must remain ultimately with the client. Many men seeking assistance with this issue will require continuing support during this process, and until a supportive network of their own can be established.

While there are support groups in the community—such as 'coming out' groups for young men, gay and married men's groups—and while these groups provide peer support and often access to other networks in the gay community, the practitioner should be aware that not every client seeking assistance will have the social skills and confidence to be able to access such groups. Rather than considering referral to a peer support group as an immediate solution, the practitioner needs to assess the client's personal resources to make links to such groups. A period of self-esteem building or personal counselling may well be a prerequisite to such a referral.

Similarly, where the client's significant others face difficulties in dealing with the client's 'new' or newly proclaimed identity, referral to support groups for parents and friends of gays, or their referral for individual or family counselling may be beneficial. While a client may hope for an outcome that preserves a hitherto positive relationship with parents and significant others, anticipating the consequences brought about by non-acceptance or open hostility is often an exigency that needs to be canvassed and planned for.

ACHIEVING INTIMACY

This term will be used to cover a variety of forms of intimate relationships between men regardless of their longevity or the many different social contexts in which they occur. Throughout their lives many gay men have the opportunity of engaging in many different forms of intimate relationships. Some of these are casual, brief, transitory and multifarious; others are permanent, long-term and exclusive. Because there are fewer formal norms for gay men's relationships, and because not all gay men choose to partner, there appears to be more opportunity for gay men to develop different kinds of intimate relationships compared with their heterosexual counterparts. This situation brings with it opportunities, but also potential challenges as personal needs are juxtaposed against dominant societal norms and institutions, many of which are unable to deal with same-sex intimacy.

Whether because there are fewer social institutions and personal and legal rituals associated with the forming and ending of personal partnerships in gay relationships (compared with the social institutions of marriage and divorce), or whether gay men have been more adventurous than their heterosexual counterparts, clinical and personal experience bears testimony to the fact that gay men form many different types of intimate relationships. Some men choose to partner. Some of those partnerships are monogamous, some 'open' or non-monogamous, and others move through different stages where rules and expectations are the subject of negotiation from time to time. With some couples the amount of sex each partner has with other men outside the relationship, and the rules under which this occurs, are varied. Other men, either in their lifetime, or for periods of it, choose to remain 'single' and satisfy their needs for intimacy with a range of brief relationships or encounters.

Since the beginning of the modern gay liberation movements there has been a renewed interest in sex and sexual expression as a form of recreation rather than necessarily tied to an intimate relationship or relationships. Such a view of sexual expression has brought challenges to fitting this behaviour to forms of intimacy. These opportunities, particularly freed from the constraints of reproduction and other heterosexual gender and social pressures, have led to a burgeoning of exploration with different partners and different expressions of sexuality (Rofes 1996). Men have been able to explore not only orthodox sexual behaviour such as intercourse and mutual masturbation, but also explore other erogenous activities associated with 'gender bending' (such as in cross-dressing) or with other forms of sexual 'play' such as in sadomasochistic, bondage and domination practices, for example. In addition, this exploration has occurred within public as well as private spaces. In the former case, a large gay sex industry has developed of clubs and merchants of retail goods and services to meet the needs of this growing diversity in sexual expression.

This diversity in sexual expression has influenced social relationships and community structures (Driggs & Finn 1991). From the clinician's viewpoint the importance of individualisation, as in the case of 'coming out' dealt with above, must be a hallmark of good practice. One of the difficulties for some gay men is dealing with the tension between establishing their own norms of behaviour as gay men, individually or in couples, and trying to mould their behaviour to the dominant norms of heterosexual orthodoxy enshrined both formally and informally in social institutions. The stages of a gay relationship have been explicated in research (McWhirter & Mattinson 1984; 1985), and it may well be useful for a couple to compare these templates with the characteristics of their own relationships. However, it is important for couples to explore their own needs and relationship patterns. Because of the relative lack of explicit history, the lack of role models, and the lack of societal templates, the challenges of living in unorthodox ways, such as in open relationships, in *ménage-à-trois*, or in households often brings additional pressures, which in some cases leads to the need for counselling (Driggs & Finn 1991).

In dealing with these situations the practitioner needs to blend training in negotiation and conflict resolution skills with education and an evaluation and/or re-affirmation of the client's value framework. Many clients find themselves trapped within an orthodoxy that can be challenged through deconstruction. It seems particularly problematic that some gay male couples resort to unsuitable templates such as the monogamous nuclear heterosexual family on which to base expectations for their own relationship and intimacy needs. This is especially salient considering that such templates are often anachronistic and hence unworkable for many contemporary heterosexual couples. In applying any technique for values clarification and conflict resolution for the construction of more suitable models, the practitioner needs to be creative in enunciating a range of possibilities in order to assist the client.

A particular challenge is assisting some clients in the process of establishing intimate relationships in the first place. While the gay community provides many types of venues and media services with a variety of options for people to socialise and to meet others, practitioners in this area will be aware of the difficulties some gay men encounter. This may reflect lack of opportunities because of geographic or social isolation, and this may be related to low levels of self-esteem and self-confidence and poorly developed skills of social negotiation. On the other hand, it may reflect a client's age or other characteristic that make it difficult to meet suitable others, and this may in part reflect the prejudices and 'isms' that are just as much part of the gay community as part of the broader community (Appleby & Anastas 1998; Roberts 2000).

COPING WITH HOMOPHOBIA

One of the key tasks for the practitioner is a consideration of the ways in which homophobia impacts upon the client and the ways in which homophobia, in its variety of forms, is part of any perceived problem (Sidoti 1999; Mason & Tomsen 1997; GLAD 1994; Wotherspoon 1991; Roberts 1989a; 1989b). As popularly used the term homophobia is an umbrella to cover a range of overt and covert discriminatory practices directed against gay men. Individual discrimination and prejudice can be directed towards gay men in the form of physical and verbal abuse, loss of opportunity and 'invisibility'. At a structural level, discrimination can take the form of non-recognition of the special needs of gay men and lack of recognition in legal and social rights that would otherwise be accorded to heterosexuals (Bluemfeld 1992; Herek 1993)

A particular form of homophobia, internalised homophobia (Bluemfeld 1992), occurs when the gay identified client takes on the same belief system and world view used to oppress gay men and applies it to himself. This usually has significant effects in lowering the person's self-esteem, assisting him to accept his position as a second-class citizen without the same rights as his heterosexual counterparts, and requiring him to decrease his visibility as a gay man. Internalised homophobia not only helps galvanise the closed closet door, but it reinforces attempts to deny any feelings that challenge the continued domination of heterosexuality.

In my experience in working with gay men it is the case that helping them confront their own internalised homophobia is often a prerequisite to helping them to deal with the homophobic actions of others. Even where anti-discrimination and anti-vilification legislation is in place, many gay men cannot access and use such legal provision to protect them where their self-esteem and their sense of being gay is weak. Prior to their being able to mobilise any action plans to stop particular forms of discrimination, or to put in place actions of recourse where physical or emotional harms have been directed towards them, there needs to be a building of their self-esteem and their self-image as citizens with the same rights as others (Garnets *et al.* 1993; Ruthchild 1997).

This can often be achieved by resorting to rational argument concerning human rights, through the use of role models and, importantly, by reference to biographical and autobiographical accounts of others' situations. Where internalised homophobia has been entrenched over a protracted period, or the stakes for coming to terms with one's difference are high, then some form of continuing psychotherapy may be required. Involving the client in community and political action groups directly, or encouraging them to read accounts of such actions, may facilitate a re-evaluation of the person's place in a socio-historical context, thus making it easier to shift one's position.

As a tool for facilitating a client's re-enactment of past experiences, reconstructing those experiences in a more positive way, and also as a vehicle for rehearsing new forms of behavioural responses, role-play, Gestalt and psycho-dramaturgical techniques have proved useful. These techniques are best employed in a group context. This provides a useful context for both experiencing changes in affect in the presence of others as well as being able to observe the experiences, reactions and solutions of others. An important precursor to behavioural change is the opportunity to rehearse situations in advance. Being able to practise responses to new, difficult and potentially harmful real-life scenarios facilitates the development of new skills and altered affects.

Establishing or renewing a client's consciousness as a gay man with rights and expectations is often challenging in those gay men who present for counselling. In my experience, while each of the challenges referred to in this chapter ('coming out', 'achieving intimacy', and 'coping with homophobia') can be observed independently of each other, they are often linked to each other in some way. Where a client has not been able to deal successfully with these aspects of his life this is frequently associated with problematic substance use, depression, low work satisfaction and isolation problems. However, the association of these behaviours with the client's sexual orientation, or a gay lifestyle, needs to be carefully assessed along with other concomitants. Just as it would be dangerous and inaccurate to assume that a client's being gay is the primary problem, so too, it is naive to underestimate the debilitating effects of entrenched, often subtle, forms of homophobia on individual people.

CONCLUSION

Human service practitioners will meet many gay men as clients in the course of their practice. Some they may not recognise as gay, and the degree to which their gay identity affects the problems they bring and the types of service they request will vary. If contemporary societies were structured differently, the sexual orientation of this client group would be unremarkable and could remain unacknowledged as a salient factor in service provision. However, ingrained homophobia and heterosexism, in all its different forms, requires that practitioners acknowledge the additional requirements of service provision that may be needed by this client group, regardless of the presenting problems.

16 | Challenging heterosexual dominance and celebrating sexual diversity in the human services

Steve Golding

The importance of understanding heterosexual dominance and homophobia was brought home to me during several workshops on these issues facilitated by a gay man who worked with men who were HIV positive. Through these workshops, I gained a greater appreciation of the role of heterosexual dominance in shaping our experience of our bodies, our sense of self and identity, our sexuality and masculinity, and our relationships with other men and women. My understanding developed further working as a sexual health counsellor in Family Planning South Australia (FPSA).[1]

In this chapter I will share some of my learning and its practical application with the intention of bringing this topic more clearly into awareness in the human services. I will explore heterosexual dominance and homophobia and why I believe it is important to understand them in our work with heterosexual men, as well as with men who identify as gay, bisexual or trans-gendered.[2] I will also outline some of the questions, dilemmas and principles in addressing these issues.

There are several important things to acknowledge in talking about this work. First, I identify as heterosexual. While this has always been so for me, and seems likely to continue to be, I understand sexuality as fluid, something that develops and changes throughout life, rather than as being fixed.

Second, other people in FPSA were also thinking about hetero-sexual dominance and homophobia. These issues were poignant to the gay, lesbian and bisexual people in the organisation who had taken various steps already to address them.

Third, in the context of this chapter, I will refer particularly to the effects of heterosexual dominance and homophobia on men and our work with men. However, heterosexual dominance and homophobia are equally important to understand and address for women who identify as lesbian, bisexual and heterosexual.

Fourth, feminist women have contributed significantly to the literature in these areas, as have men and women identifying as gay, lesbian, bisexual and trans-gendered. Relatively little of the ideas and analysis at this point in history comes from heterosexually identified men (Connell & Dowsett 1993; Hollway 1996; Rich-ardson 1996).

WHAT ARE HETEROSEXUAL DOMINANCE AND HOMOPHOBIA?

Heterosexuality is one of the definers of privilege and power in our culture. Evidence of this confronts us every day. The media is populated with images of happy heterosexual sex, relationships, couples and families. Some men are bashed or murdered in city parklands even for looking like they might be gay. It was only in 1996 that the Australian Bureau of Statistics Census recognised same-sex partners for the first time. This was a notable step forward that also highlighted the barriers to recognition of same-sex rela-tionships. Furthermore, until recently there were still laws against same-sex relationships and sexual practices in one Australian state.

Heterosexual dominance is a form of historical, cultural, insti-tutional and social oppression. It involves access to power and privilege for those who identify or are seen as heterosexual and its denial to those who identify or are perceived as being outside the dominant culture by virtue of their sexual identification. The dominant culture of heterosexuality is promoted by major social institutions, and all other sexualities are simultaneously subordi-nated. Heterosexual dominance thus involves discrimination and prejudice. When our institutions and organisations perpetuate these injustices and act on them, heterosexual dominance is at work. Within a culture of heterosexual dominance, our primary frame of reference comes from a heterosexual perspective, and attitudes, services and resources are oriented to recognise and engage pro-actively with heterosexuality.

The dominant or hegemonic (Connell 1995) culture of hetero-sexuality also promotes the belief that one pattern of relationships and sexual intimacy is naturally superior to all others. Other possibilities are not acknowledged, or are actively undermined. This is oppressive and abusive to men who identify as gay and bisexual and is very confining for men who identify as heterosexual.

Homophobia is a direct outcome of living in a culture of heterosexual dominance and it plays a role in maintaining and perpetuating it. Homophobia can be experienced in a range of ways including: fear of lesbians and gay men; fear of feeling love or attraction for members of one's own sex and therefore the hatred of those feelings in others; dislike for people based on their sexuality; or fear of being perceived as not being heterosexual.

To focus on homophobia in isolation from heterosexual domi-nance is problematic as it situates the 'problem' of a 'phobic response' individually rather than within the broader politics of power and privilege (Hopkins 1992). This limited focus supports oppression by psychologising and individualising structural issues.[3]

HETEROSEXUAL DOMINANCE AND INVISIBILITY

Dominance is often invisible to members of the dominant group, while it is often painfully obvious for members of the oppressed group. Gay and bisexual men may be left in a position of having to argue to heterosexual people that their oppression exists. Hetero-sexuals may have difficulty taking this seriously because it does not reflect their experience. This invisibility may show itself in human service organisations by heterosexual staff not seeing heterosexual dominance and homophobia as issues of relevance to their work.

Heterosexual people might say things like: 'We treat people equally regardless of sexuality.' 'Why is a person's sexuality an issue anyway? Can't we all just be people?' 'If you'd just stop thinking about yourself as oppressed and get on with it, it'd all be OK.' 'Why are you so sensitive?' 'Why do you have to make such a big deal about your sexuality anyway?'

People and organisations can replicate heterosexual dominance without necessarily being homophobic. An agency may treat gay or bisexual men respectfully, if they present for service, without opening space which challenges the dominant culture. They may not make it clear that sexualities, other than heterosexuality, are welcomed, supported and celebrated. A heterosexual person may not hold homophobic attitudes and may treat gay and bisexual men with respect, without recognising that they are still a heterosexual person in a culture and society where that gives them privilege whether they like it or not and whether they personally feel privileged or not. For example, simply being free and safe to walk down the street holding hands with your partner is a privilege not shared equally between heterosexual partners and same-sex partners. A heterosexual person may not appreciate the impact of living with this and many other such instances on a daily basis and may not see their greater freedom and safety as one aspect of privilege within a culture of dominance. Heterosexual people do not have to think about what it means to be heterosexual while gay and bisexual men have to put considerable thought into this.

Language is one important issue in representing or failing to represent the interests of individuals and groups, in making visible or keeping invisible their lives and experience, and in challenging or participating in and perpetuating the dominant culture. Literature on 'manhood' that is really about 'heterosexual manhood' reproduces heterosexual dominance by treating heterosexual masculinity as if it represents all masculinity while totally or largely failing to make visible the diverse sexualities of men. In this context, silence on the part of mainstream human service organisations, or people identifying as heterosexual, becomes collusion—a passive maintenance of dominance by failing to acknowledge those marginalised by the dominant culture.

WHY IS UNDERSTANDING HETEROSEXUAL DOMINANCE IMPORTANT?

I believe it is essential for people working in the human services to explicitly recognise and address heterosexual dominance and homophobia in their work with men for three main reasons. First, heterosexual dominance and homophobia are issues of social justice, equal opportunity and human rights. Second, heterosexual dominance and homophobia affect us all through their role in the social construction of masculinity, relationships and sexuality. Third, we need to understand these forms of dominance and their effects, in order to be able to explicitly recognise and appropriately respond to the needs of men who have same-sex sexual relationships.

Heterosexual dominance and homophobia interrupt men's ability to express sexual diversity safely and actively create risk for people who express sexuality that is different from the accepted norm. This generates a range of barriers to access to information and services, which make it harder to maintain and improve health and wellbeing. It also interferes with people's freedom to enjoy their sexuality and relationships.

HOW DO HETEROSEXUAL DOMINANCE AND HOMOPHOBIA HURT US ALL?

Heterosexual dominance and homophobia actively oppress men who identify as gay or bisexual. They also have effects in the lives of men who identify as heterosexual. For example, they inhibit the freedom of heterosexual men to form close, intimate relationships with other men for fear of being perceived as gay. They contribute to rigid masculine roles that inhibit creativity and self-expression. They inhibit freedom to express our human traits and diverse ways of being a man (Miller & Mahamati 1994). Heterosexual models for sexual relationships that emphasise 'attraction of opposites', may tend to blind us to possibilities for sexual relationships of equality and similarity (Richardson 1996).

Addressing heterosexual dominance and homophobia is an issue of rights for gay and bisexual men. It also recognises that heterosexual dominance frames all of our work with men and is central to understanding sexuality and masculinity. By challenging heterosexual dominance and homophobia, we address the oppression of specific groups of men, and contribute to a society that accepts and celebrates the differences in us all.

A FRAMEWORK FOR RESPONDING TO HETEROSEXUAL DOMINANCE

One starting place is to analyse heterosexual dominance with a scale such as that developed by Riddle (cited in Miller & Mahamati 1994). She suggested repulsion, pity, tolerance and acceptance as four main homophobic attitudes. These are not used to suggest objective 'levels of homophobia', but as a way to think about attitudes that inform, feed and reflect it. They reflect externalisation of oppression, as they are directed outwardly towards others.

Table 1   Scale of Attitudes

	Internalised Oppression: attitudes and self-evaluation	Externalised Oppression: attitudes and expression to others
Subject to the effects of heterosexual dominance	Self-hatred Self-pity Resignation	Repulsion Pity Tolerance
Dealing with the effects of heterosexual dominance	Self-acceptance Self-love Supportiveness	Acceptance Support Admiration
Challenging heterosexual dominance	Pride Celebration	Appreciation Nurturance/Celebration

Riddle also suggested support, admiration, appreciation and nurturance as four positive attitudes towards homosexuality.

Miller and Mahamati (1994) suggest a similar scale, arranging internalised negative attitudes towards homosexuality into three areas of self-hatred, self-pity and resignation. They suggest another three attitudes that reflect dealing with homophobia as self-acceptance, self-love and supportiveness. Two further attitudes they suggest as transcending homophobia are pride and celebration.

I have adapted and combined these two scales in Table 1 to capture some of the negative and damaging effects of heterosexual dominance on attitudes and personal experience, together with some of the positive and beneficial effects of challenging heterosexual dominance. I prefer celebration to nurturance as a term in Riddle's scale to avoid any patronising overtones.

These scales can be applied to any form of dominance and oppression and can be explored at the personal or organisational level. There are problems inherent in the use of such scales. Their use can imply a progression from 'bad' to 'better' to 'good' attitudes. The element of judgment in this is not helpful in promoting open discussion and exploration. Scales may suggest being at just one point, but you can be at different places on different issues at the same time. For example, a man may think and feel quite differently about hugging close male friends than he does about the thought of two men having sex together.

A number of themes and questions can be developed from these scales as tools for evaluating the degree to which social work practices or human service organisations reflect or challenge heterosexual dominance and homophobia. Outcomes of this evaluation provide a basis for strategic planning and action to challenge heterosexual dominance and homophobia.

In Figure 1 I have organised a number of questions into a framework to facilitate recognising these issues and devising strategies to address them in our service provision with men.

Figure 1   Framework for analysing heterosexual dominance

Section A: Is it recognised as a problem?

1. How could it be established whether the way programs and services have been provided in relation to the issues of heterosexual dominance and homophobia are a problem?
2. What are key questions in addressing these issues and devising strategies?
3. How could developmental goals and practical strategies in thinking and practice be established?
4. What would these goals be?

Section B: How does the service rate?

1. Where might the agency be on the scale of externalised oppression in relation to gay or bisexual men?
2. What might be the experience of a gay or bisexual man coming into the agency?
3. What might be the experience of a gay or bisexual man working in the agency?
4. How might staff speak and think about the life and relationships of a gay or bisexual colleague, if they knew of his sexuality?
5. Do gay or bisexual staff feel safe to talk about their everyday lives with colleagues?
6. How might first-hand information from gay or bisexual men and from key organisations serving these communities be obtained?

Section C: Accountability

1. How does the organisation acknowledge the issue of dominance and recognise the need for accountability?
2. Is it recognised that people from the culture of dominance whose experience is more of privilege are less likely to recognise oppression and the experience of oppression than people who experience it directly?
3. What might that mean for practices, processes and principles of accountability?

Section D: Agency responsibility

1. What do the agency mandate, mission and goals, and staff and management beliefs about people, relationships and sexuality, suggest about how the agency might need to develop?
2. If the agency were at a point of appreciation and nurturance of sexual diversity, of recognising this as a human rights issue, and encouraging pride and celebration, how might that be shown?

3.   Are gay or bisexual issues seen as primarily the 'personal agenda' of certain staff members?
4.   If so why?
5.   What might it reflect about the influence of heterosexual dominance if this is the case?

Section E: Policy and planning

1.   How do organisational policy and planning support addressing heterosexual dominance and responding to the needs of gay or bisexual men?
2.   Are there written policy and strategic planning documents which provide a clear framework for acknowledging and addressing heterosexual dominance as an integral part of the activities of the organisation?
3.   Do job and person specifications reflect a need for awareness of the issues created by heterosexual dominance?

Section F: Advocacy and leadership

1.   How does the organisation respond to public expressions of homophobia? Is silence collusive?
2.   In light of the mission and goals of the organisation, what are its advocacy and leadership roles, as well as its service provision roles?
3.   For a person struggling with issues relating to their sexuality, what changes in the environment would support this person to feel more able to celebrate their sexuality?

Section G: Resources

1.   Excluding HIV/AIDS related projects, what resources does the organisation put towards programs and services for gay or bisexual men and communities?
2.   What acknowledgment is made of the possible numbers of gay or bisexual workers and clients?
3.   How well do agency programs and services address the sexuality and needs of gay or bisexual men?

Section H: Agency networks

1.   What relationship does the agency have with other agencies that address the issues of gay or bisexual men?
2.   What attempts have been made to establish formal links?
3.   What are the blocks to establishing such links?
4.   Are any links largely informal, existing because particular gay or bisexual staff have created them?

Section I: Visibility

1.   What messages do the general promotional material of the organisation contain about gay and bisexual men and relationships?
2.   Are there visual images of men of diverse sexualities? Is written and spoken language inclusive of these communities?
3.   Are gay and bisexual men named as part of the target population?
4.   When heterosexual masculinity or sexuality are mentioned, are they identified explicitly as heterosexual, or are they referred to generically, as if

masculinity and sexuality are heterosexual and anything else is a special add-on case?

5. Does the organisation have easily accessible materials addressing gay and bisexual issues other than HIV?

Section J: Training and education

1. Does training offered by the organisation address the effects of heterosexual dominance on its communities of interest?
2. Does training acknowledge the effects of heterosexual dominance and homophobia on men identifying as heterosexual as well as on gay and bisexual men?
3. Does training recognise how it benefits heterosexual men to challenge heterosexual dominance and homophobia as well as how it benefits gay and bisexual men?
4. What are the roles and responsibilities of educators in raising and challenging heterosexual dominance and homophobia?

Section K: Vulnerability

1. What might it mean for a gay or bisexual man to be part of discussions about heterosexual dominance and homophobia as a staff member?
2. Do people of the dominant group make themselves vulnerable in talking about their lives and experience in trying to come to terms with these issues?
3. What does the organisation do to ensure the occupational health and safety of gay or bisexual workers who face homophobia in carrying out their daily role?

Section L: Worker–client communication

1. Is it okay for workers to reveal their sexuality to clients?
2. What happens when clients reveal their sexuality?

CHALLENGING HETEROSEXUAL DOMINANCE IN FAMILY PLANNING SOUTH AUSTRALIA

The issues and questions raised in this chapter can be applied broadly to human service organisations and social work practice. The following example relates these issues and questions to the service provision, planning and policy of FPSA as a mainstream sexual health service.

FPSA began as a family planning and reproductive health service at a time when homosexuality was illegal in South Australia. Historically it provided mainly clinical services primarily to white, middle-class women. For several years prior to 1995, FPSA reviewed its work and shifted focus from family planning to sexual health adopting the principles of social justice and primary health care as its basis for planning and service delivery.

FPSA's broad mission statement (FPSA 1994) was to enable people to:

- express their sexuality safely;
- maintain and improve their sexual health; and
- enjoy their sexuality.

This was not a 'heterosexual mission'. It did not exclude people who identified as gay, lesbian, bisexual or trans-gendered. For example, FPSA's organisational values statement included 'valuing diversity'. However, it was not active inclusion, but a passive intention. In a culture of dominance, individuals and organisations must go beyond passive 'inclusion by default' to active inclusion to challenge the patterns of erasure.[4]

Breaking the silence by starting more open discussion about heterosexual dominance and homophobia, what they mean in our work and what they mean in people's lives, challenges heterosexual dominance. What does not challenge dominant culture, supports it by default and supports the maintenance of structures of privilege and power that have real effects in the lives, relationships and experience of people who are marginalised.

In 1995 I initiated conversation within FPSA about heterosexual dominance and homophobia. I thought it was important, as a man identifying as heterosexual, to facilitate this discussion in the organisation. I believe it would have been replicating heterosexual dominance to leave it only to gay, lesbian or bisexual people to raise the issues.

The strategic plan and organisational mission and goals developed in line with FPSA's change of focus provided a context that supported and legitimised, and even actively required these issues to be recognised and addressed. FPSA began to explore how to move from having good intentions, and a few key staff 'championing' the rights of people who identified as gay, lesbian, bisexual and trans-gendered, to having a visible, proactive approach integral to the whole organisation.

As I am committed to principles of accountability and partnership in addressing issues of dominance, my next step was discussion with all those who were 'out' as gay, lesbian or bisexual in the organisation. This focused on sharing my motivation for raising the issues, emphasising the importance of the process being one of partnership accountability, and exploring any concerns and hopes they had for the process and its outcomes.

A timely discussion paper on these issues was published (White 1995), making clear information easily available. At the team level, management support was quickly gained and planning how to develop discussion of these issues across the organisation began.

Articles from the discussion paper were circulated to all teams. I followed this up by discussion with team leaders in each team and with the people who were 'out' as gay, lesbian or bisexual about the processes for facilitating discussion at the team level. The management team were included in this as they were keen to discuss the issues and participate in the process, with some specific focus on management responsibility in relation to these issues.

Clearly, management support was important. Individual time with the Chief Executive Officer (CEO) focused on the importance of these issues and of having organisational space for discussion. The CEO saw this fitting clearly with the strategic directions and wanted to see policy outcomes—a process to get heterosexual dominance and the needs of gay, lesbian, bisexual and trans-gendered people onto the agenda for the whole organisation as well as documentation of the process and outcomes.

I facilitated discussion in all teams. All staff had the opportunity and invitation to participate in discussion of the issues and their relevance to us. One prime goal in the team discussion process was to open a safe space for people to talk about heterosexual dominance and homophobia and begin to explore in open conversation what they meant for our work on issues of social justice, equal opportunity and human rights. The intention was for developmental discussion at all levels rather than top-down policy imposition.

A second goal was to achieve some shared understanding of heterosexual dominance and homophobia—what they are, how they work, and how they affect our lives. Also, for each team to begin to recognise collectively the relevance of heterosexual dominance and homophobia to our work.

A third goal was to identify next steps for the organisation. We discussed questions such as whether it was important for FPSA, as a specialist sexual health agency and the major sexual health organisation for the state, to have explicit reference in organisational policy and strategic planning to the needs of gay, lesbian, bisexual and trans-gender communities.

DILEMMAS AND PRINCIPLES IN CHALLENGING
HETEROSEXUAL DOMINANCE

From my participation in leading this process I was able to identify some of the principles and dilemmas that are important to consider in such work. Changes by members of a dominant group that involve some response to correct social injustice must involve a process of accountability in order to address the imbalance of power. Accountability must be to those subject to the injustice so that their experience informs the process of change. This involves accepting responsibility not just for our actions and for their direct effects, but also for recognising our membership of groups that bestow privilege and power on us. It is also important for a person in a dominant group who opens up discussion of these issues to do so from a position that recognises that they have a lot to learn, and not to see themself as a crusader or as occupying the moral high ground compared to other heterosexual people.

Raising these issues can be an isolating experience for the person organising the discussions. To have these issues discussed will be uncomfortable for many people and there may be elements of 'backlash'. There is potential for division because many of us (particularly those of us with membership in dominant groups) are not used to open discussion about issues of dominance and oppression in which we situate ourselves and where people with membership in dominant groups are confronted with privilege and its effects. It may elicit homophobic responses and the person organising the discussion may experience aspects of gay oppression. It is also important for us to learn how to discuss such issues in ways that free us from a sense of guilt, blame or polarisation so that we can change.

It is often easy to find strategies and solutions and to focus on the practicalities of 'what we have to do to make things different'. However, there are also other things that are important to talk about along the way. To talk openly and talk through some of the hard issues about heterosexual dominance before entering into strategy and action is in itself a radical step and a challenge to heterosexual dominance.

For a heterosexual person choosing to initiate discussion in these areas, it is important to be prepared to see it through—even if it takes time and energy and gets harder than expected. This is an issue of accountability. Consider what it could mean for people who identify as gay, lesbian, bisexual or trans-gendered in the organisation, firstly for the discussion to be raised, and secondly if it were dropped because it got too hard for the person who raised it. Part of heterosexual privilege includes being able to walk away from the issue because it is not part of one's everyday life and experience in the way that it is if one is a member of a marginalised group.

CONCLUSION

While in the past we might have thought that the main issues facing men were heterosexual masculinity and male–female relationships, it is time to step back and see how this view is framed by heterosexual dominance. This view does not allow us to recognise the fullness of masculinity or of men's sexuality—only of a constrained heterosexual masculinity. It leaves out the lives and experiences of many men. This has negative effects for the work we do, and for those whom we serve.

To suggest greater freedom to explore sexual relationships, sexual identity and sexual practices, as derived from broader non-discriminatory frameworks, does not suggest any pressure on any person to move in any direction they do not wish to. It does, however, suggest a richer, more informed, approach that opens more possibilities for exploring non-exploitative and equality-based sexual relationships.

I believe that failure to take up the issue of explicitly valuing sexual diversity in human service organisations reflects a failure to support human rights, and a failure to promote health, wellbeing and equitable access to services for all.[5]

Endnotes

CHAPTER 1

1 See, for example, Brook and Davis (1985); Marchant and Wearing (1986); Hanmer and Statham (1988); Dominelli and McLeod (1989); Taylor (1990); Langan and Day (1992) and Weeks (1994).
2 See Cavanagh and Cree (1996).
3 See, for example, Ife (1997); Mullaly (1997); Thompson (1998).
4 In the Australian context see, for example, Connell (1995); Buchbinder (1998) and Peterson (1999).
5 Again, in the Australian context, see Biddulph (1994); Edgar (1997) and Morton (1997).
6 See, for example, Huggins *et al.* (1996); Camer-Pesci (1997); Commonwealth Department of Human Services and Health (1997) and South Australian Health Commission (1997).
7 In 1998 the Commonwealth Attorney General's Department organised a national forum on Men and Family Relationships attended by over 500 professionals working with men. They also made available $6 million for services aimed at working with men in families. See National Forum on Men and Family Relationships (1998).
8 The Commonwealth Government recently released a report on policy responses to the funding of groups for violent men. See Report to National Crime Prevention (1999).
9 See, for example, Kenway and Willis (1997); Gilbert and Gilbert (1999) and Lingard and Douglas (1999).

10 See, for example, Polk (1994); Newburn and Stanko (1994) and Collier (1998).
11 See Pease (1998) for a more extensive discussion of these different approaches.
12 The main intellectual sources of the men's rights movement can be found in the work of Baumli (1985); Lyndon (1992); Farrell (1993) and Thomas (1993).
13 See Pease (1995) for a detailed account of the origins and activities of Men Against Sexual Assault.

CHAPTER 2

1 See, for example, Taubman (1986); Meth and Pasick (1990) and Brooks (1998). For a critique of the limitations of sex role analysis in men's health promotion, see Pease (1999a).
2 I am currently working on an international, cross-cultural writing project eliciting accounts of men's practices in ten countries, including India, Hong Kong, Brazil, Nicaragua and South Africa, as well as five Western countries, a way of both contextualising and globalising men's subjectivities and practices. See Pease and Pringle (forthcoming).
3 A researcher's standpoint 'emerges from one's social position with respect to gender, culture, colour, ethnicity, class and sexual orientation and the way in which these factors interact and affect one's everyday world' (Swigonski 1993, p. 172).
4 May (1998) refers to a progressive male standpoint to elucidate this perspective. There is also a parallel here with the development of anti-racism. White people can develop a sufficient understanding of racism to adopt a white anti-racist standpoint. See, for example, Frankenberg (1993).
5 See, for example, Kimmel and Mosmiller (1992) for a documentary history of profeminist men's work in the United States from 1776–1990.
6 For a detailed analysis of the implications of postmodernism for theorising men, see Pease (2000).
7 See Pease (1999b) for an account of men using an anti-sexist consciousness-raising group to understand their own sexist behaviour.

CHAPTER 7

1 The quotes used in this chapter form part of my PhD research.
2 Hegemonic masculinity is the dominance of a set of normalised 'attributes and rules against which other masculine practices are

measured' (Jewitt 1997, p. 2.3). Connell (1995, p. 77) states that these practices act to legitimise patriarchy in order to maintain dominance.

3 Research into female perpetrators has revealed higher incidence rates than first thought (Peluso and Putnam 1996).

4 CASA (1998) found that females had a greater vulnerability to sexual violence throughout their lifecycle compared to men. Although this does not take into account the high rate of sexual assault in correctional facilities that have very high populations of males (see Heilpern 1998).

5 See North American Man/Boy Love Association (NAMBLA), see Cermak and Molidor (1996, p. 397).

6 Initial studies into the prevalence of sexual abuse of children purported that male victims were a very small minority of the victims (Finkelhor 1984). Nasjleti (1980) in her research found that male children were largely unrecognised victims of sexual violence, and this prompted her to suggest many male victims go on to 'suffer in silence'.

7 This forms part of my PhD research.

8 These introductory and practice ideas are expanded upon in O'Leary (1998).

9 My research found also that males and females were likely to get an inadequate response if they disclosed abuse at the time.

CHAPTER 10

1 This chapter is derived from a presentation to the Justice and Change: Creating Integrated and Coordinated Criminal Justice Responses to Family and Domestic Violence in Australia Conference, Canberra. September 29–1 October 1999. I would like to thank Dallas Colley, Jennifer MacKenzie, the women of WOWSafe, David Jones, Alison Newton and Alan Jenkins for commenting upon earlier drafts of this chapter.

CHAPTER 14

1 This conversation took place in Melbourne in January 2000.

2 This was our tribal boundary prior to European occupation and like Eddie Mabo the Yorta Yorta argued that our native title rights had survived the tide of European settlement. None of my ancestors ever ceded or signed their native title rights to the colonial government who appropriated most of this land.

3 Kitty Atkinson/Cooper's mother, Mariah, was born at the Moira Lakes before 1788.

4 See Ian Clark (1990).

5 Edward Stone Parker was the Chief Protector for the Loddon Aboriginal Protectorate.

6 Formerly known as the Victorian Aboriginal Child Placement Agency it changed its name to Victorian Aboriginal Child Care Agency (VACCA) in late 1977.

7 See Judy Atkinson (1990).

8 Atkinson (1990) uses the term emasculation for describing this process.

CHAPTER 15

1 Throughout the chapter I use the terms 'gay identified men' and 'gay men' (or the singular form) interchangeably. This is my attempt to emphasise an adjectival quality, rather than a noun-like quality. By doing so, I hope to avoid an essentialist approach to 'being gay'. For a useful discussion on essentialism versus social constructionism the reader should refer to Altman et al. (1989).

2 The terms 'gender' and 'sexual orientation' will be used in this chapter in conventional form. The reader should refer to Masters, Johnson and Kolodny (1988) and Allgeier and Allgeier (1988) for a fuller explication of these concepts. For an applied use, see Pronger (1990).

3 While male homosexuality has now been decriminalised in all Australian states and territories and some states have enacted anti-discrimination and anti-vilification legislation with reference to gay men and lesbians, considerable change is still required to ensure that gay men and lesbians have access to the same rights and obligations as their heterosexual counterparts, for example, in same-sex marriage, parenting, superannuation rights and so on.

4 As this is a book about men, I will use the masculine pronoun throughout the chapter. In no way is this meant to challenge the principle of non-sexist language in other respects.

5 The class 'men who have sex with men' (MSM) was developed by researchers interested in observing behaviours separated from a particular sexual identity. The separation of MSM and gay men appeared in research on the transmission of HIV where the actual behaviours were significant irrespective of sexual orientation. See, for example, Dowsett (1990) and Roberts (1994).

CHAPTER 16

1 Formerly FPSA, now SHINE (Sexual Health Information Networking and Education) SA.

2 For ease of writing I will refer to men who identify as gay or bisexual when talking about the diverse range of sexualities marginalised by the dominant culture of heterosexuality. This itself is a limited description of the diversity of men's sexuality.

3 There is a wealth of literature that explores the nature of and connections between heterosexual dominance, homophobia, masculinity and sexuality including Connell and Dowsett (1993); Kimmel (1997); and Richardson (1996).

4 Erasure here refers to the processes of making invisible the existence, lives and experiences of gay, lesbian, bisexual or trans-gender people.

5 A number of people at FPSA contributed significantly to the process and inspired the development of the ideas and thinking in this chapter. I want to particularly acknowledge my long-term friend and colleague Jen Hamer, and Sally Gibson, who both contributed to conference presentations of some of this work in partnership around gender and sexuality. Thanks to Leanne Black, Ralph Brew, Bev Burnell, Jacq Hackett, John McKiernan, Kerry Telford, and Kaisu Vartto. Thanks also to Chris McLean, who edited an earlier draft of this chapter.

Bibliography

ABS 1997 *Suicide Prevention Victorian Task Force Report* Australian Bureau of Statistics, Canberra.

ABS 1999 *Prisoners in Australia* 1998 Australian Bureau of Statistics, Commonwealth of Australia, Canberra.

Adams, R.G. 1994 'Older men's friendship patterns' *Older Men's Lives* ed. E. Thompson Jnr, Sage, Thousand Oaks, CA.

Alcoff, L. and Gray, L. 1993 'Survivor discourse: Transgression or recuperation?' *Signs: Journal of Women in Culture and Society* vol. 18, no. 2, pp. 260–89.

Allen, J. and Gordan, S. 1990 'Creating a framework for change' *Men in Therapy* eds R. Meth & R. Pasick, The Guilford Press, New York.

Allgeier, A.R. and Allgeier, E.R. 1988 *Sexual Interactions* Heath & Co, Lexington, Massachusetts.

Altman, D., Vance, C., Vicinus, M. and Weeks, J. 1989 *Homosexuality, Which Homosexuality?* Gay Men's Press, London.

Anderson, A. 1998 'Strengths of gay male youth: An untold story' *Journal of Child and Adolescent Social Work* vol. 15, no. 1 pp. 55–71.

Anderson, H. and Goolishian, H. 1988 'Human systems as linguistic systems: Preliminary and evolving ideas about the implications for clinical theory' *Family Process* vol. 27, no. 4, pp. 371–94.

Appleby, G. and Anastas, J. 1998 *Not Just A Passing Phase: Social Work with Gay, Lesbian and Bisexual People* Columbia University Press, New York.

Applegate, J.S. 1997 'Theorising older men' *Elderly Men: Special Problems and Professional Challenges* eds J. Kosberg & L. Kaye, Springer, New York.

Atkinson, J. 1990 'Violence against Aboriginal women: Reconstitution of community law' *Aboriginal Law Bulletin* vol. 2, pp. 6–9.

Australian Association of Social Workers 1999 *Code of Ethics* AASW, Canberra.

Australian Bureau of Statistics 1996 *Community Service Australia 1995–6* ABS, Canberra.

Babbit, S. 1993 'Feminism and objective interests: The role of transformative experiences in rational deliberation' *Feminist Epistemologies* eds L. Alcoff & E. Potter, Routledge, New York.

Ball, G. 1997 'A Psychopathology of Everyday Masculinity' Unpublished Masters Thesis, La Trobe University, School of English, Melbourne.

Baltes, P. and Baltes, M. 1990 *Successful Ageing: Perspectives from the Behavioral Sciences* Cambridge University Press, New York.

Barer, B.M. 1994 'Men and women aging differently' *The International Journal of Aging and Human Development* 38, pp. 29–40.

Barkam, M 1992 'Research on integrative and eclectic therapy' *Integrative and Eclectic Therapy: A Handbook* ed. W. Dryden, Open University Press, Milton Keynes.

Barusch, A. and Peak, T. 1997 'Support groups for older men: Building on strengths and facilitating relationships' *Elderly Men: Special Problems and Professional Challenges* eds J. Kosberg & L. Kaye, Springer, New York.

Bateson, G. 1973 *Steps to an Ecology of Mind* London, Paladin.

Bathrick, D. and Kaufman, G. 1990 'Male privilege and male violence: Patriarchy's root and branch' *Men and Intimacy* ed. F. Abbott, The Crossing Press, Freedon CA.

Baumli, F. ed. 1985 *Men Freeing Men* New Atlantic Press, Jersey City.

Bazemore, G. and Walgrove, I. eds 1999 *Restorative Juvenile Justice* Criminal Justice Press, New York.

Beckett, S. 1936 *Murphy* London, Routledge.

Belsky, J. and Cassidy, J. 1996 'Attachment: Theory and evidence' *Development Through Life; A Handbook for Clinicians* eds M. Rutter & D.F. Hay. Blackwell, Oxford.

Bengston, V., Rosenthal, C. and Burton, L. 1996 'Paradoxes of families and aging' *Handbook of Aging and the Social Sciences* eds R. Binstock & L. George, Academic Press, San Diego, CA.

Bengston, V., Burgess, E. and Parrott, T. 1997 'Theory, Explanation and a Third Generation of Theoretical Development in Social Gerontology' *Journal of Gerontology* vol. 28, no. 2, pp. S72–S88.

Berger, R and Kelly, J 1986, 'Working with homosexuals in the older population' *Social Casework* no. 67, pp. 203–10.

Berger, R. 1982 *Gay and Gray: The Older Homosexual Man* University of Illinois Press, Urbana, Ill.

Berkman, C. and Zinberg, G. 1997 'Homophobia and heterosexism in social workers' *Social Work* vol. 42, no. 4, pp. 319–32.

Biddulph, S. 1994 *Manhood* Finch, Sydney.

Biles, D. Harding, R. Walker, J. 1999 *The Deaths of Offenders Serving Community Corrections Orders* Trends and Issues in Crime and Criminal Justice no. 107, Australian Institute of Criminology, Canberra.

Bliss, S. 1986 'Beyond machismo: The new men's movement' *Yoga Journal* (November/December), pp. 36–40, 57–8.

Blumenfeld, W. ed. 1992 *Homophobia: How we all Pay the Price* Beacon Press, Boston.

Bly, R. 1987a 'What men really want: Interview with Keith Thompson' *New Men, New Minds* ed. F. Abbott, The Crossing Press, Freedom. CA.

Bly, R. 1990 *Iron John: A Book About Men* Addison Wesley, New York.

Borowski, A. 1990 'Older workers and the work-leisure choice: The causes of early retirement in Australia' *Australian Social Work* vol. 43, no. 2, pp. 27–36.

Borowski, A., Encel, S. and Ozanne, E. eds 1997 *Ageing and Social Policy in Australia* Cambridge University Press, Melbourne.

Bowlby, J. 1958 'The nature of a child's tie to his mother' *International Journal of Psychoanalysis* vol. 39, pp. 350–73.

Boyd-Franklin, N., Franklin, A. 1999 'African-American couples in therapy' *Revisioning Family Therapy: Race, Culture, and Gender in Clinical Practice* ed. M. McGoldrick, Guildford, New York.

Braithwaite, J. and Daly, K. 1994 'Masculinities and communitarian control' *Just Boys Doing Business? Men, masculinities and Crime* eds T. Newburn & E. Stanko, Routledge, London.

Briggs, F. 1995 *From Victim to Offender, How Child Sexual Abuse Victims Become Offenders* Allen & Unwin, Sydney.

Briggs, F., Hawkins, R.M.F. and Williams, M. 1994 A comparison of the early childhood and family experiences of incarcerated, convicted male child molesters and men who were sexually abused in childhood and have no convictions for sexual offences against children, University of South Australia, Magill Campus, South Australia.

Brod, H. 1998 'To be a man or not to be a man: That is the feminist question' *Men Doing Feminism* ed. T. Rigby, Routledge, New York.

Brook, E and Davis, A. eds 1985 *Women, the Family and Social Work* Tavistock, London.

Brooks, G. 1991 'Traditional men in marital and family therapy' *Feminist Approaches for Men in Family Therapy* ed. M. Bograd, Haworth Press, New York.

Brooks, G. 1998 *A New Psychotherapy for Traditional Men* Jossey-Bass, San Francisco.

Bryson, L. 1992 *Welfare and the State* Macmillan, London.

Buchbinder, D. 1994 *Masculinities and Identities* Melbourne, Melbourne University Press.

Buchbinder, D. 1998 *Performance Anxieties: Re-Producing Masculinity* Allen & Unwin, Sydney.

Buckley, K. 1996 'Masculinity, the probation service and causes of offending behaviour' *Working with Offenders: Issues, Contexts and Outcomes* eds T. May & A. Vass, Sage, London.

Burns, G. 1998 'A perspective on policy and practice in the re-integration of offenders' *European Journal on Criminal Policy and Research* no. 6, pp. 171–83.

Calam, R., Horne, L., Glasgow, D. and Cox, A. 1998 'Psychological disturbance and child sexual abuse: A follow-up study' *Child Abuse and Neglect* vol. 22, no. 9, pp. 901–13.

Camer-Pesci, P. 1997 *Men's Health Policy: A Discussion Paper* Health Department of Western Australia.

Camilleri, P. 1996 *(Re)Constructing Social Work* Avebury, Aldershot.

Carr, A., 1998 'The inclusion of fathers in family therapy: A research based perspective' *Contemporary Family Therapy* vol. 20, no. 3, September, pp. 371–83.

CASA (Centre Against Sexual Assault) 1998 'Phone in Against Sexual Assault September 1998' unpublished paper, Melbourne.

Cass, V. C. 1979 'Homosexual identity formation: A theoretical model' *Journal of Homosexuality* vol. 4, pp. 219–35.

Cavanagh, K. and Cree, V. eds 1996 *Working With Men: Feminism and Social Work* Routledge, London.

Cecchin, G. and Lane, G. 1993 'From strategizing to non-intervention: Towards irreverence in systemic practice' *Journal of Marital and Family Therapy* vol. 19, no. 2, pp. 125–36.

Cermak, P. and Molidor, C. 1996 'Male victims of child sexual abuse' *Child and Adolescent Social Work Journal* vol. 13, no. 5, pp. 385–400.

Chandy, J.M., Blum, R.W. and Resnick, M.D. 1996 'Gender-specific outcomes for sexually abused adolescents' *Child Abuse and Neglect* vol. 20, no. 12, pp. 1219–31.

Chaplin, J 1988 *Feminist Counselling in Action* Sage, London.

Chodorow, N. 1978 *The Reproduction of Mothering* University of California Press, Berkeley.

Christie, A. 1998 'Is social work a "non-traditional" occupation for men?' *British Journal of Social Work* vol. 28, pp. 491–510.

Clark, I. 1990 *Aboriginal Language and Clans: An Historical Atlas of Western and Central Victoria, 1800–1900* Monash Publications, Melbourne.

Clinical Evaluation Review Team 1994 *Clinical Evaluation of the Vietnam Veterans Counselling Service* Clinical Evaluation Review Team, Vietnam Veterans' Counselling Service, Melbourne.

Cockburn, C. 1988 Contributor to roundtable discussion, 'Mending the broken heart of socialism' *Male Order: Unwrapping Masculinity* eds R. Chapman & J. Rutherford, Lawrence and Wishart, London.

Cockburn, C. 1991 *In The Way of Women* Macmillan, London.

Coleman, E. 1985 'Developmental stages of the coming out process' *A Guide to Psychotherapy with Gay and Lesbian Clients* ed. J.C. Gonsiorek, Harrington Park Press, New York.

Coles, R. 1997 *The Moral Intelligence of Children* Bloomsbury, London.

Colley, D. 1991 'What's a nice woman like me doing in a place like this?' *Dulwich Centre Newsletter* no. 1, pp. 26–7.

Colley, D., Hall, R., Jenkins, A., and Anderson, G. 1997 *Competency Standards for Intervention Workers Working with Men who Perpetrate Domestic Abuse and Violence* The Office for Families and Children, Adelaide.

Collier, R. 1998 *Masculinities, Crime and Criminology* Sage, London.

Collinson, D. 1992 *Managing The Shopfloor: Subjectivity, Masculinity and Workplace Culture* de Gruyter, Berlin.

Commonwealth Department of Health, Housing, Local Government and Community Services 1993 *Aged Care Reform Strategy Mid Term Review* Stage 2 Australian Government Publishing Service, Canberra.

Commonwealth Department of Human Services and Health 1997 Draft National Men's Health Policy Primary Health Care Group, Canberra.

Commonwealth Department of Veterans Affairs 1998 *Veterans At Risk* Research Project undertaken by Thomson Goodall Associates, Canberra.

Connell, R.W. 1987 *Gender and Power* Polity Press, Cambridge.

Connell, R. W. 1991 'The big picture—A little sketch: changing western masculinities in the perspective of recent world history' Paper presented at the Research on Masculinity and Men in Gender Relations Conference, Sydney, 7–8 June.

Connell, R. W. 1992 'Drumming up the wrong tree' *Tikkun* vol. 7, no. 1, pp. 31–6.

Connell, R.W. 1995 *Masculinities* Allen & Unwin, Sydney

Connell, R.W. and Dowsett, G. 1993 'Introduction' *Rethinking Sex: Social Theory and Sexuality Research* eds R.W. Connell & G.W. Dowsett, Temple University Press, Philadelphia.

Cox, G. 1990 *The Streetwatch Report: A Study into Violence Against Lesbians and Gay Men* Gay and Lesbian Rights Lobby of New South Wales, Sydney.

Cox, G. 1994 *The Count and Counter Report; A Study into Hate Related Violence Against Lesbians and Gay Men* Gay and Lesbian Rights Lobby of New South Wales, Sydney.

Davies, B. 1989 *Frogs and Snails and Feminist Tales* Allen & Unwin, Sydney.

Davies, B. and Harre, R. 1990 'Positioning: The discursive production of selves' *Journal for the Theory of Social Behaviour* vol. 20, no. 1, pp. 43–63.

Deinhart, A., and Myers-Avis, J., 1994 'Working with men in family therapy: An exploratory study *Family Process* vol. 20, no. 4, October, pp. 397–418.

Dempsey, K. 1997 *Inequalities in Marriage* Oxford University Press, Melbourne.

Department of Employment, Education and Training 1991 *Australia's Workforce in the Year 2001* Australian Government Publishing Service, Canberra.

Department of Justice 1999 Weekly Community Correctional Services Report I, 1999

(Unpublished data) compiled by the Office of Correctional Services, Victorian Department of Justice.

DeVore, I. and Owen Lovejoy, C. 1985 'The natural superiority of women' *The Physical and Mental Health of Aged Women* eds M. Haug, A. Ford & M. Shaefor, Springer, New York.

Dhaliwal, G.K., Gauzas, L., Antonowicz, D.H. and Ross, R.R. 1996 'Adult male survivors of childhood sexual abuse: Prevalence, sexual abuse characteristics, and long-term effects' *Clinical Psychology Review* vol. 16, no. 7, pp. 619–39.

Dienhart, S. and Myers-Avis, J. 1994 'Working with men in family therapy' *Family Process* vol. 20, no. 4, pp. 387–418.

Dolan-DelVeccio, K. 1998 'Dismantling white male privilege within family therapy' *Revisioning Family Therapy: Race, Culture, and Gender in Clinical Practice* ed. M. McGoldrick, Guildford, New York.

Dominelli, L. and McLeod, E. 1989 *Feminist Social Work* Macmillan, London.

Donovan Research 1999 *Men's Counselling Research* Attorney General's Department, Canberra.

Douglas, P. 1993 'Men = Violence: A profeminist perspective on dismantling the masculine equation' Paper presented at the Second National Confernece on Violence, Canberra, Australian Institute of Criminology.

Dowsett G. 1990 'Reaching men who have sex with men in Australia' *Australian Journal of Social Issues*, vol. 25, no. 3, pp. 186–98.

Driggs, J. and Finn, S. 1991 *Intimacy Between Men* Plume Books, New York.

Dunlop, B., Rothman, M. and Rambali, C. 1997 'Elderly men in retirement communities' *Elderly Men: Special Problems and Professional Challenges* eds J. Kosberg & L. Kaye, Springer, New York.

Dutton, D., 1995 'Male abusiveness in intimate relationships' *Clinical Psychology Review* vol. 15, no. 6, pp. 567–81.

Edgar, D. 1997 *Men, Mateship, Marriage* Harper Collins, Melbourne.

Edley, N. and Wetherell, M. 1995 *Men in Perspective: Practice, Power and Identity* Prentice Hall, London.

Egan, G. 1997 *The Skilled Helper* 5th edition, Pacific Grove, Brooks-Cole.

Egeland B., Jacobvitz D. and Sroufe L. 1988 'Breaking the cycle of abuse: Relationship predictors' *Child Development* vol. 59, pp. 1080–88.

Eisler, R. and Loye, D. 1990 *The Partnership Way* Harper, San Francisco.

Erikson, E., Erikson, J. and H. Kivnick 1986 *Vital Involvement in Old Age: The Experience of Old Age in Our Time* Norton and Company, New York.

Eysenck, H. 1952 'The Effects of Psychotherapy: An Evaluation' *Journal Of Consulting Psychology* vol. 16, pp. 319–24.

Family Planning South Australia 1994 *Strategic Directions 1994/95 to 1996/97* Adelaide.

Faria, G. 1997 'The challenge of health care social work with gay men and lesbians' *Social Work in Health Care* vol. 25, no. 1, pp. 65–72.

Farkas, K. and Kola, L. 1997 'Recognizing and treating alcohol abuse and alcohol dependence in elderly men' *Elderly Men: Special Problems and Professional Challenges* eds J. Kosberg & L. Kaye, Springer, New York.

Farmer, S. 1991 *The Wounded Male* Ballantine, New York.

Farrell, W. 1975 *The Liberated Man* Bantam, New York.

Farrell, W. 1993 *The Myth of Male Power* Simon and Schuster, New York.

Federal Bureau of Prisons 1997 *State of the Bureau* Federal Bureau of Prisons, United States of America.

Finch, J. and Groves, D. eds 1983 *A Labour of Love: Women, Work and Caring* Routledge and Kegan Paul, London.

Finkelhor, D. 1984 *Child Sexual Abuse: New Theory and Research* Free Press, New York.

Finkelhor, D. Hotaling, G. Lewis, I.A. Smith, C. 1990 'Sexual abuse in a national survey of adult men and women: Prevalence characteristics and risk factors' *Child Abuse and Neglect* vol. 14, pp. 19–28.

Finkelhor, D. and Browne, A. 1985 'The traumatic impact of child sexual abuse: A conceptualization' *American Journal of Orthopsychiatry* vol. 55, no. 4, pp. 530–41.

Fletcher, R., 1999 Report of the Men and Boys Project of the Family Action Centre, The University of Newcastle.

Fonagy, P. 1997 'Morality, disruptive behaviour, borderline personality disorder, crime and their relationships to security of attachment' *Attachment and Psychopathology*, eds L. Atkinson & K. Zuker, Guilford, New York.

Fondacaro, K.M., Holt, J.C. and Powell, T.A. 1999 'Psychological impact of childhood sexual abuse on male inmates: The importance of perception' *Child Abuse and Neglect* vol. 23, no. 4, pp. 361–9.

Foucault, M 1967 *Madness and Civilisation: A History of Insanity in the Age of Reason* Tavistock, London.

Francis, J. Linke, P. and Castell McGregor, S. 1995 *To Hit or Not to Hit: The Question of Physical Punishment of Children: A Practical Guide for Parents about Discipline* Children's Interest Bureau, Adelaide

Frankenberg, R. 1993 *White Women, Race Matters: The Social Construction of Whiteness* Routledge, London.

Furlong, M. 1995 'Difference, indifference and differentiation' *Australian and New Zealand Journal of Family Therapy* vol. 16, no. 1, pp. 15–22.

Furlong, M. 1996 'Cross purposes: Emotional patterns in child welfare' *The Therapeutic Relationship in Systemic Practice* eds C. Flaskas & A. Perlesz, Karnac Books, London.

Furlong, M. 1997 'Sports stories: The metaphors of sport for the game of life' *Arena* no. 31, pp. 39–42.

Furlong, M. And Lipp, J. 1995 'The multiple relationships between neutrality and therapeutic influence' *Australian and New Zealand Journal of Family Therapy*, vol. 16, no. 4, pp. 201–11.

Gallagher-Thompson, D. and Osgood, N. 1997 'Suicide in later life' *Behavior Therapy* vol. 28, pp. 23–41.

Ganley, A. 1990 'Feminist therapy with male clients' *Feminist Approaches For Men in Family Therapy* ed. M. Bograd, Haworth Press, New York.

Garbarino, J. 1999 *Lost Boys* Free Press, New York.

Gardner, I., Brooke, E., Ozanne, E. and Kendig, H. 1998 *Improving Social Networks: A Research Report* Commonwealth Department of Veterans Affairs, Canberra.

Garnets L. and Kimmel, D. eds 1993 *Psychological Perspectives on Lesbian and Gay Male Experiences* Columbia University Press, New York.

Garnets, L. and Kimmel, D. 1993 'Lesbian and gay male dimensions in the psychological study of human diversity' *Psychological Perspectives on Lesbian and Gay Male Experiences* eds L. Garnets & D. Kimmel, Columbia University Press, New York.

Garnets, L. Herek, G. and Levy, B. 1993 'Violence and victimisation of lesbians and gay men: Mental health consequences' *Psychological Perspectives on Lesbian and Gay Male Experiences* eds L. Garnets & D. Kimmel, Columbia University Press, New York.

Gay Men and Lesbians Against Discrimination 1994 *Not a Day Goes By* Report on the GLAD Survey into Discrimination and Violence Against Lesbians and Gay Men in Victoria, Melbourne.

Gibelman, M. and Schervish, P. 1995 'Pay equity in Social Work: Not!' *Social Work* vol. 40, no. 5, pp. 622–9.

Gilbert, R. and Gilbert, P. 1999 *Masculinity Goes to School* Allen & Unwin, Sydney.

Gill, M. and Tutty, L.M. 1997 'Sexual identity issues for male survivors of childhood sexual abuse: A qualitative study' *Journal of Child Sexual Abuse* vol. 6, no. 3, pp. 31–47.

Gill, M. and Tutty, L.M. 1999 'Male survivors of childhood sexual abuse: A qualitative study and issues for clinical consideration' *Journal of Child Sexual Abuse* vol. 7, no. 3, pp. 19–33.

Gilligan, C. 1982 *In a Different Voice* Harvard University Press, Cambridge.

Gilmore, D 1990 *Manhood in the Making* Yale University Press, London.

Goldberg, H. 1987 *The Inner Male* Signet, New York.

Goldman, J.D.G. and Padayachi, U.K. 1997 'The prevalence and nature of child sexual abuse in Queensland, Australia' *Child Abuse and Neglect,* vol. 21, no. 5, pp. 489–98.

Goldner, V. 1991 'Toward a critical relational theory of gender' *Psychoanalytic Dialogues* vol. 1, no. 3, pp. 249–72.

Goldner, V. 1992 'Making room for both/and' *Family Therapy Networker* vol. 16, no. 2.

Goldner, V. 1995 'Boys will be men: A response to Terry Real's paper' *Journal of Feminist Family Therapy* vol. 7, nos. 1/2, pp. 45–48.

Goldner, V. 1998 'The treatment of violence and victimization in intimate relationships' *Family Process* vol. 37, no. 3.

Goldner, V. Penn, P. , Sheinberg, N., and Walker, G., 1990 'Love and violence: Gender paradoxes in volatile attachments' *Family Process* vol. 29, no. 4, pp. 343–64.

Goldscheider, F. 1990 'The aging of the gender revolution' *Research on Aging* vol. 12, no. 14, pp. 531–45.

Goldstein, H. 1983 'Starting where the client is' *Social Casework* May, pp. 267–75.

Gomez, J. 1991 *Psychological and Psychiatric Problems in Men* Routledge, London.

Gonyea, J. 1994 'Making gender visible in public policy' *Older Men's Lives* ed. E. Thompson Jr., Sage, Thousand Oaks, CA.

Gottman, J. 1994 *Why Marriages Succeed or Fail* Simon and Schuster, New York.

Gradman, T. 1994 'Masculine identity from work to retirement' *Older Men's Lives* ed. E. Thompson Jr., Sage, Thousand Oaks, CA.

Graham, H. 1983 'Caring: A labour of love' *A Labour of Love: Women, Work and Caring* eds J. Finch and D. Groves, Routledge and Kegan Paul, London.

Greenberg, D.F. 1988 *The Construction of Homosexuality* University of Chicago Press, Chicago

Guillemard, A-M. 1993 'Older workers and the labour market' *Older People in Europe: Social and Economic Policies* eds A. Walker, J. Alber & A. Guillemard, Commission of the European Communities.

Guisinger, S. and Blatt, S. 1994 'Individuality and relatedness' *American Psychologist* vol. 49, no. 2, pp. 104–11.

Gutmann, D. 1987 *Reclaimed Powers: Toward a New Psychology of Men and Women in Later Life* Basic Books, New York.

Gutmann, D. and Huyck M. 1994 'Development and pathology in postparental men: A community study' *Older Men's Lives* ed. E. Thompson Jr, Sage, Thousand Oaks, CA.

Hall, W. 1995 'Substance Abuse' *Men and Mental Health* ed. A. Jorm, National Health and Medical Research Council, Australian Government Publishing Service, Canberra.

Hamilton, G. 1940 *Theory and Practice of Social Casework* Columbia University Press, New York.

Hanmer, J. and Statham, D. 1988 *Women and Social Work: Towards a Woman Centred Practice* Macmillan, London.

Hare-Mustin R.T. and Marecek J. 1986 'Autonomy and gender: Some questions for therapists' *Psychotherapy* vol. 23, no. 2, pp. 205–12.

Harre, R. and Vanlangenhove, L. 1991 'Varieties of positioning' *Journal for the Theory of Social Behaviour* vol. 21, no. 4, pp. 393–406.

Harrison, J. 1997 'Social policy and Aboriginal people' *Ageing and Social Policy in Australia* eds A. Borowski, S. Encel & E. Ozanne, Cambridge University Press, Melbourne.

Haug, M., Ford, A., and Shaefor, M. 1985 *The Physical and Mental Health of Aged Women* Springer, New York.

Hayward, M., Piental, A., McLaughlin, D. 1997 'Inequality in men's mortality: The socioeconomic status gradient and geographic context' *Journal of Health and Social Behavior* vol. 38, no. 4, pp. 313–30.

Hearn, J. 1987 *The Gender of Oppression: Men Masculinity and the Critique of Marxism* Wheatsheath, Sussex.

Hearn, J. 1992 *Men in the Public Eye* Routledge, London.

Hearn, J. 1999 'It's time for men to change' *Working With Men For Change* ed. J. Wild, UCL Press, London.

Heath, V., Bean, R. and Feinauer, L. 1996 'Severity of childhood sexual abuse: Symptom differences between men and women' *The American Journal of Family Therapy* vol. 24, no. 4, pp. 305–14.

Heelas, P. and Lock, A. 1981 *Indigenous Psychologies: An Anthropology of the Self* Academic Press, London.

Heilpern, D. 1998 *Fear or Favour: Sexual Assault of Young Prisoners* Southern Cross University Press, New South Wales.

Herek, G. 1993 'The context of anti-gay violence: Notes on cultural and psychological heterosexism' *Psychological Perspectives on Lesbian and Gay Male Experiences* eds L. Garnets & D. Kimmel, Columbia University Press, New York.

Herrman H., McGarry, P., Mills, J. and Singh, B. 1991 'Hidden severe psychiatric morbidity in sentenced prisoners: An Australian study' *American Journal of Psychiatry*, vol. 148, no. 2, pp. 236–9.

Hershberger, S. Pilkington, N. and D'Augelli, A. 1997 'Predictors of suicide attempts among gay, lesbian and bisexual youth' *Journal of Adolescent Research* vol. 12, no. 4, pp. 477–97.

Hollway, W. 1996 'Recognition and Heterosexual Desire' *Theorising Heterosexuality* ed. D. Richardson, Open University Press, Philadelphia.

Holmes, G.R., Offen, L. and Waller, G. 1997 'See no evil, hear no evil, speak no evil: Why do relatively few male victims of childhood sexual abuse receive help for abuse-related issues in adulthood?' *Clinical Psychology Review* vol. 17, no. 1, pp. 69–88.

hooks, b. 1992 *Black Looks: Race and Representation* South End Press, Boston.

Hooyman, N., and Kiyak, H. 1996 *Social Gerontology, A Multidisiçplinary Perspective* Allyn and Bacon, Boston.

Hopkins, P. 1992 'Gender Treachery: Homophobia, Masculinity, and Threatened Identities' *Rethinking Masculinity: Philosophical Explorations in Light of Feminism* eds L. May & R.A. Strikwerda with the assistance of P. Hopkins, Littlefield Adams Quality paperbacks, Maryland.

Horst, E., and Doherty, W.J. 1995 'Gender, power and intimacy' *Journal of Feminist Family Therapy* vol. 6, pp. 63–85.

Howe, D. 1986 'The segregation of women and their work in the personal social services' *Critical Social Policy* vol. 15, pp. 21–36.

Howells, K. and Day, A. 1999 'The Rehabilitation of Offenders: International Perspectives Applied to Australian Correctional Systems' *Trends and Issues in Crime and Criminal Justice*, no. 112, Australian Institute of Criminology, Canberra.

Huber, R. and Orlando, B. 1995 'Persisting gender differences in social workers' incomes: Does the profession really care?' *Social Work* vol. 40, no. 5, pp. 585–91.

Hudson, A 1988 'Boys will be boys: Masculinism and the juvenile justice system' *Critical Social Policy* no. 21.

Hudson, J., Morris, M. and Gallaway, B. 1996 *Family Group Conferences* Federation Press, Sydney.

Huggins, A., Somerford, P. and Rouse, I. 1996 *A Report on Men's Health* Western Australia, School of Public Health, Curtin University, Perth.

Hugman, R. 1991 *Power in Caring Professions* Macmillan, London.

Hunter, J.A. Jr., Goodwin, D.W. and Wilson, R.J. 1992 'Attributions of blame in child sexual abuse victims: An analysis of age and gender influences' *Journal of Child Sexual Abuse* vol. 1, no. 3, pp. 75–89.

Husaini, B. 1997 'Predictors of depression among the elderly: Racial differences over time' *American Journal of Orthopsychiatry* vol. 67, no. 1, pp. 48–58.

Ife, J. 1997 *Rethinking Social Work: Towards Critical Practice* Longman, Melbourne.

Isparo, A.J. 1986 'Male client–male therapist: Issues in a therapeutic alliance' *Psychotherapy* vol. 23, pp. 257–66.

Jablensky, A., McGrath, J., Hermann, H., Castle, D., Gureje, O., Morgan, V. and Korten, A. 1999 *People Living with Psychotic Illness: An Australian Study* National Survey of Mental Health and Wellbeing, Report 4, National Mental Health Strategy, Department of Health and Aged Care, Canberra.

Jackson, D. 1990 *Unmasking Masculinity: A Critical Biography* Unwin Hyman, London.

James, K. 1983 'Breaking the chains of gender: Family therapy's position?' *Australian Journal of Family Therapy* vol. 5, no. 4, pp. 236–44.

James, K. 1999 Securing the bases: The implications of attachment theory for parenting boys and working with men in therapy *Relationships into the New Millennium* Papers to Celebrate 50 years of Relationships Australia, Relationships Australia, Canberra.

Jefferson, T. 1994 'Theorising masculine subjectivity' *Just Boys Doing Business? Men, Masculinities and Crime* eds T. Newburn & E. Stanko, Routledge, London.

Jenkins, A. 1990 *Invitations to Responsibility. The Therapeutic Engagement of Men Who are Violent and Abusive* Dulwich Centre Publications, Adelaide.

Jewitt, C. 1997 'Images of men: Male sexuality in sexual health leaflets and posters for young people' *Sociological Research Online* vol. 2, no. 2, http://www.socresonline.org.uk/socresonline/2/2/6.html.

Jimenez, M. 1997 'Gender and psychiatry: Psychiatric conceptions of mental disorders in women, 1960–1994' *Affilia: Journal of Women and Social Work* vol. 12, pp. 154–75.

Johnson, D. 1996 'The developmental experience of gay/lesbian youth' *Journal of College Admission* Summer/Fall Edn pp. 38–41.

Jones, E. 1993 *Family Systems Therapy, Developments in the Milan-Systemic Therapies* John Wiley and Sons, London.

Jones, E. 1995 'The construction of gender in family therapy' *Gender, Power and Relationships* ed. C. Burck & B. Speed, Routledge, London.

Jukes, A. 1993 *Why Men Hate Women* Free Association Books, London.

Kaufman, M. 1993 *Cracking The Armour: Power, Pain and the Lives of Men* Viking, Toronto.

Keen, S. 1991 *Fire in the Belly: On Being a Man* Bantam Books, New York.

Kelly, L., Burton, S. and Regan, L. 1994 'Researching women's lives or studying women's oppression? Reflections on what constitutes feminist research' *Researching Women's Lives From a Feminist Perspective* eds M. Maynard and J. Purvis, Taylor & Francis, London.

Kenway, J. and Willis, S. 1997 *Answering Back: Girls, Boys and Feminism in Schools* Allen & Unwin, Sydney.

Kimmel, M. 1994 'Masculinity as homophobia' *Theorizing Masculinities* eds H. Brod & M. Kaufman, Sage, London.

Kimmel, M. and Messner, M. 1989 'Introduction' *Men's Lives* eds M. Kimmel & M. Messner, Macmillan, New York.

Kimmel, M. and Messner, M. eds 1992 *Men's Lives* 2nd edn, Macmillan, New York.

Kimmel, M. and Mosmiller, T. 1992 eds *Against the Tide: Profeminist Men in the United States 1776–1990* Beacon Press, Boston.

Kindlon, D. and Thompson, M. 1999 *Raising Cain: Protecting the Emotional Life of Boys* Ballantine Books, New York.

King, B. 1992 'The men's movement' *Arena* nos. 99/100, pp. 129–40.

Kipnis, A 1999 *Angry Young Men* Jossey Bass, San Francisco.

Knox, J. 1996 'A prison perspective' *Working With Men* eds K. Cavanagh & V. Cree, Routledge, London.

Knudson-Martin, C., and Mahoney, A. 1999 'Beyond different worlds: A "post gender" approach to relational development' *Family Process* vol. 30, no. 3, pp. 325–40.

Kosberg, J. and Bowie S. 1997 'The victimization of elderly men' *Elderly Men: Special Problems and Professional Challenges* eds J. Kosberg & L. Kaye, Springer, New York.

Kosberg, J. and Kaye, L. 1997 'The status of older men: Current perspectives and future projections' *Elderly Men: Special Problems and Professional Challenges* eds J. Kosberg & L. Kaye, Springer, New York.

Kreiner, C. 1992 'Giving up sexism' *The Liberation of Men* Rational Island Publisers, Seattle.

Krout, J., McCulloch, B. and Kivett, V. 1997 'Rural older men: A neglected elderly population' *Elderly Men: Special Problems and Professional Challenges* eds J. Kosberg & L. Kaye, Springer, New York.

Kupers, T. 1993 *Revisioning Men's Lives: Gender, Intimacy and Power* The Guilford Press, New York.

Langon, M. and Day, L. eds 1992 *Women, Oppression and Social Wants* Routledge, London.

Lau, A. 1995 'Gender, power and relationships: Ethno-cultural and religious issues' *Gender, Power and Relationships* ed. C. Burck & B. Speed, Routledge, London.

Lawrence, J. 1965 *Professional Social Work in Australia* Australian National University Press, Canberra.

Lawton, M. and Nahemow, L. 1973 'Ecology and the aging process' *Psychology of Adult Development and Aging* eds C. Eisdorfer & M. Lawton, American Psychological Association, Washington D.C.

Lawton, M.P. 1983 'Environment and other determinants of well-being in older people' *The Gerontologist* vol. 23, pp. 349–57.

Lee, J. 1991 *At My Father's Wedding: Reclaiming Our True Masculinity* Bantam, New York.

Leonard, P. and Nichols, B. eds 1994 *Gender, Aging and the State* Blackrose Books, Montreal.

Lerner, G. 1986 *The Creation of Patriarchy* Oxford University Press, New York.

Lesbian and Gay Community Action of South Australia 1994 *The Police and You* LGCASA, Adelaide.

Levinson, D. 1989 *Family Violence in Cross Cultural Perspective* Sage, Newbury Park, CA.

Levinson, D., Darrow, C., Klein, E., Levinson, M. and McKee, B. 1978 *The Seasons of a Man's Life* Knopf, New York.

Lew, M., 1990 *Victims No Longer: A Guide for Men Recovering from Sexual Child Abuse* Mandarin Paperbacks, London.

Lewis, Myrna 1985 'Older women and health: An overview of health needs of women as they age' *Women and Health* vol. 10, no. 2/3, pp. 38–49.

Lingard, B. and Douglas, P. 1999 *Men Engaging Feminisms: Pro-feminism, Backlashes and Schooling* Open University Press, Buckingham.

Longres, J. 1995 *Human Behaviour in the Social Environment* Peacock Publishers, Itasca.

Lowe, R. 1990 'Re-imagining family therapy: Choosing the metaphors we live by' *Australian and New Zealand Journal of Family Therapy* vol. 11, no. 1, pp. 1–10.

Lyndon, N. 1992 *No More Sex War: The Failures of Feminism.* Sinclair-Stevenson, London.

McGuire, J. 1995 *What Works Reducing Recidivism* John Viney.

McIntosh, J., Pearson, J. and Lebowitz, B. 1997 'Mental disorders of elderly men' *Elderly Men: Special Problems and Professional Challenges* eds J. Kosberg & L. Kaye, Springer, New York.

McIntosh, J., Santos, J., Hubbard, R. and Overholser, J. 1994 *Elder Suicide: Research, Theory and Treatment* American Psychological Association, Washington D.C.

MacKinnon, L. 1998 *Trust and Betrayal in the Treatment of Child Abuse* Guildford, New York.

McWhirter, D. and Mattinson, A. 1985 'Psychotherapy for gay male couples' *A Guide to Psychotherapy with Gay and Lesbian Clients* ed. J. Gonsiorek, Harrington Park Press, New York.

McWhirter, D.P. and Mattison, A.M. 1984 *The Male Couple: How Relationships Develop* Prentice-Hall, Englewood Cliffs, New Jersey.

MaCold, P. 1997 *Restorative Justice: An Annotated Bibliography* Criminal Justice Press, New York.

Mahdi, L., Foster S. and Little M. 1987 *Betwixt and Between* Open Court Publishing, La Salle, Illinois.

Mallon, G. 1994 'Counseling strategies with gay and lesbian youth' *Helping Gay and Lesbian Youth* ed. T. DeCrescenzo, Harrington Park Press, Binghamton.

Mangum, W. 1997 'A demographic overview of elderly men' *Elderly Men: Special Problems and Professional Challenges* J. Kosberg & L. Kaye, Springer, New York.

Marchant, H. and Wearing, B. eds 1986 *Gender Reclaimed: Women in Social Work* Hale and Iremonger, Sydney

Martin, E 1996 'An update on census data: Good news for social work?' *Australian Social Work* vol. 49, no. 2, pp. 29–36.

Martin, E. 1990 Gender, demand and domain: The social work profession in South Australia 1935–1980, PhD Thesis, Melbourne University, Melbourne.

Martin, E. and Healy, J. 1993 'Social work as women's work: Census data 1976–1986' *Australian Journal of Social Work* vol. 46, no. 4, pp. 13–18.

Mason, G. and Tomsen, S. eds. 1997 *Homophobic Violence* Hawkins Press, Sydney.

Masters, W.H. Johnson, V.E. and Kolodny, R.C. 1988 *Human Sexuality* Scott Foresman and Co., Glenview, Illinois.

Masterson, 1988 *Search for the Real Self* The Free Press, New York.

Mathers, C. 1994 *Health Differentials Among Older Australians* Health Monitoring Series No. 2, Australian Institute of Health and Welfare, Australian Government Publishing Services, Canberra.

Matras, J. 1990 *Dependency, Obligation and Entitlement: Towards a New Sociology for Ageing, the Life Course and the Elderly* Prentice Hall, New Jersey.

May, L. 1998 'A progressive male standpoint' *Men Doing Feminism* ed. T. Digby, Routledge, New York.

Mayer, J. and Timms, N. 1969 'Clash of perspectives between worker and client' *Social Casework* vol. 50, pp. 32–40.

Mazioli, E. and Alexander, L. 1991 'The power of the therapeutic relationship' *American Journal of Orthopsychiaty* vol. 61, no. 3, pp. 383–91.

Mederos, F. 1987 'Patriarchy and male psychology' Unpublished manuscript, Montreal.

Mendel, M.P. 1995 *The Male Survivor, The Impact of Sexual Abuse* Sage, Newberry Park, CA.

Mens-Verhulst J. van 1993 'Beyond daughtering and mothering' *Daughtering and Mothering: Female Subjectivity Reanalysed* eds J. van Mens-Verhulst, K. Schreurs & L. Woertman, Routledge, London.

Meth, R. and Pasick, R. eds 1990 *Men in Therapy* Guilford Press, New York.

Middleton, P. 1992 *The Inward Gaze: Masculinity and Subjectivity in Modern Culture* Routledge, London.

Miller, A., 1983 *The Drama of the Gifted Child and the Search for the True Self* Faber and Faber, London.

Miller, B., and Cafasso, L. 1992 'Gender differences in caregiving: Fact or artifact?' *The Gerontologist* vol. 32, no. 4, pp. 498–507.

Miller, K.P. and Mahamati 1994 *'Blockout': Challenging Homophobia Education Manual* The Youth Sector Training Council (YSTC of South Australia and the Second Storey Youth Health Service.

Minton, H. and McDonald, G. 1985 'Homosexual identity formation as a developmental process' *Origins of Sexuality and Homosexuality* eds J. De Cecco & M. Shively, Harrington Park Press, New York.

Monk, A. 1981 'Social work with the aged: Principles of practice' *Social Work* vol. 61, pp. 61–8.

Moore, R. and Gillette, D. 1990 *King, Warrior, Magician, Lover: Rediscovering the Archetypes of the Mature Masculine* Harper, New York.

Morgan, M. 1992 'Therapist gender and psychoanalytic couples therapy' *Sexual and Marital Therapy* vol. 7, no. 2, pp. 141–56.

Morton, T. 1997 *Altered Mates: The Man Question* Allen & Unwin, Sydney.

Mullaly, B. 1997 *Structural Social Work: Ideology, Theory and Practice* Oxford University Press, Toronto.

Murphy, K. 1996 'Men and offending groups' *Working With Men* eds T. Newburn & G. Mair, Russell House Publishing, Dorset.

Nasjleti, M. 1980 'Suffering in silence: The male incest victim' *Child Welfare* vol. 59, no. 5, pp. 269–75.

National Inquiry into the Separation of Aboriginal and Torres Strait Islander Children from their Families (Australia) 1997 *Bringing them Home: Report of the National Inquiry into the Separation of Aboriginal and Torres Strait Islander Children from their Families* HREOC, Sydney.

National Forum on Men and Family Relationships 1998, Commonwealth Department of Family and Community Services, Canerra.

NCADA 1994 *Alcohol Misuse and Violence Report 1* Australian Government Publishing Service, Canberra.

New South Wales Police Service 1995 *Out of the Blue: A Police Survey of Violence and Harassment Against Gay Men and Lesbians* New South Wales Police Service and Price Waterhouse, Urwick, Sydney.

Newburn, T. and Stanko, A. 1994 'Introduction: Men, masculinity and

crime' *Just Boys Doing Business? Men, Masculinities and Crime* eds
T. Newburn & E. Stanko, Routledge, London.

Newburn, T. and Stanko, A. eds 1994 *Just Boys Doing Business? Men
Masculinities and Crime* Routledge, London.

Newman, S 1997 'Men's bodies, masculinities and nursing' *The Body in
Nursing* ed. M. Turpin, Churchill Livingston. Melbourne.

Neysmith S. ed. 1999 *Critical Issues for Future Social Work Practice with Aging
Persons* Columbia University Press, New York.

Northern Metropolitan Community Health Service 1997 *Stopping Violence
Groups: A Model of Best Practice for Group Work with Men Who Wish to
Stop Violent and Abusive Behaviour Toward Their Women Partners and
Family* Northern Metropolitan Community Health Service, Adelaide.

O'Brien, M. 1988 'Men and fathers in therapy' *Journal of Family Therapy*
vol. 10, pp. 109–23.

O'Hagan, K. 1997 'The problem of engaging men in child protection work'
British Journal of Social Work vol. 27, pp. 25–42.

OCSC 1999 *Statistical Profile of the Victorian Prison System 1995–96 to 1997–98*
Office of the Correctional Services Commissioner (OCSC), Department
of Justice Victoria, Melbourne.

O'Leary, P. 1998 'Liberation from self-blame: Working with men who have
experienced childhood sexual abuse' *Dulwich Centre Journal* Dulwich
Centre Publications, Adelaide, no. 4, pp. 24–40.

O'Leary, P. 1999 'Reflections on weaving new stories over the phone: An
invitation into complexities' *Gecko* Dulwich Centre Publications,
Adelaide, vol. 3, pp. 51–55.

Orkin, G. 1991 'Abuse, violence, counselling' *XY: Men, Sex, Politics* vol. 1,
no. 3, (Springer, pp. 9–11.

Orlinsky, D. Grave, D. and Parks, B. 1994 'Process and outcome in
psychotherapy' *Handbook of Psychotherapy and Behaviour Change* eds
A. Bergen and S. Garfield, 4th edn Wiley, New York.

Ozanne, E 1994 'Social work and the psychiatry of late life' *Functional
Psychiatric Disorders of the Elderly* eds E. Chiu & D. Ames, Cambridge
University Press, Cambridge.

Parsons, T and Bales, R.F. 1955 *Family, Socialization and Interaction Process*
Free Press, Glencoe, Ill.

Partnerships Against Domestic Violence 1999 *Working With Men Who Perpetrate Domestic Violence and Abuse* Comptency Standards, Adelaide.

Pasick, R. 1992 *Awakening From the Deep Sleep* Harper, San Francisco.

Paterson, T. 1996 'Leaving well alone: A systemic perspective on the
therapeutic relationship' *The Therapeutic Relationship in Systemic Practice*
eds C. Flaskas & A. Perlesz, Karnac Books, London.

Paulsen, M. 1999 'Deconstructing hegenomic masculinity' *Youth Studies
Australia* vol. 18, no. 3, pp. 12–17.

PDAC. 1996 *Drugs In Our Community* Report of the Premiers' Drug Advisory
Council, Victorian Government, Melbourne.

Pease, B. 1995 'MASA: Men against sexual assault' *Issues Facing Australian Families* eds W. Weeks and J. Wilson, 2nd edn, Longman Cheshire, Melbourne.

Pease, B 1997 *Men and Sexual Politics: Towards a Profeminist Practice* Dulwich Centre Publications, Adelaide.

Pease, B. 1998 'Dividing lines: The politics of the men's movement' *Community Quarterly* no. 47, pp. 77–88.

Pease, B. 1999a 'The politics of men's health promotion' *Just Policy* vol. 15, April, pp. 29–35.

Pease, B. 1999b 'Profeminist subjectivities: Working on the contradictions' *Mattoid: Journal of Literary and Cultural Studies* no. 54, pp. 259–73.

Pease, B 1999c 'Deconstructing masculinity—reconstructing men' *Transforming Social Work Practice* eds. B. Pease & J. Fook, Allen & Unwin, Sydney.

Pease, B. 2000 *Recreating Men: Postmodern Masculinity Politics* Sage, London.

Pease, B. and Fook J. eds 1999 *Transforming Social Work Practice: Postmodern Critical Perspectives* Allen & Unwin, Sydney.

Pease, B. and Pringle, K. eds (forthcoming) *Globalising Men: Cross-Cultural Perspectives on Men's Politics and Practices* Zed Books, London.

Peluso, E. and Putnam, N. 1996 'Case study: Sexual abuse of boys by females' *Journal of the American Academy of Child Adolescent Psychiatry* vol. 35, no. 1, pp. 51–5.

Pence, E. and Paymar, M. 1993 *Education Groups For Men Who Batter* Springer, New York.

Pepenski, H. 1998 'Making peace with our childhood' *The Justice Professional* vol. 11, pp. 159–74.

Perry B.D., Pollard R.A., Blakey T.L., Baker W.L. and Vigilante D. 1995 'Childhood trauma, the neurobiology of adaption, and "use-dependent" development of the brain: How "states" become "traits"' *Infant Mental Health Journal* vol. 16, no. 4, pp. 271–91.

Peterson, A. 1999 *Unmasking the Masculine: 'Men' and 'Identity' in a Sceptical Age* London, Sage.

Phillips, A. 1993 *The Trouble with Boys, Parenting the Men of the Future* Pandora, London.

Phillipson, C. 1996 *Capitalism and the Social Construction of Old Age* Macmillan, London.

Pithouse, A. 1987 *Social Work: The Social Organisation of an Invisible Trade* Avebury, Aldershot.

Polk, K. and White, R. 1999 'Economic adversity and criminal behaviour: Rethinking youth unemployment and crime' *Australian and New Zealand Journal of Criminology* vol. 32, no. 3 pp. 284–302.

Polk, K. 1994 *When Men Kill: Scenarios of Masculine Violence* Cambridge University Press, Cambridge.

Pollack, W. 1998 *Real Boys, Rescuing Our Sons from the Myths of Boyhood* Random House, New York.

Pollack, W., and Levant, B. 1998 *New Psychotherapy for Men* Wiley, New York.

Pringle, K 1995 *Men, Masculinities and Social Welfare* UCL Press, London.

Pringle, K. 1998 'Current profeminist debates regarding men and social welfare: Some national and transnational perspectives' *British Journal of Social Work* vol. 28, pp. 623–33.

Pronger, B. 1990 *The Arena of Masculinity: Sports, Homosexuality, and the Meaning of Sex* GMP Publishers, London.

Quinn, J. 1999 'Shifts in early exit phenomena of older men in the United States' Paper given at MIT, October, Cambridge, Mass.

Rabin, C. 1996 *Equal Partners—Good Friends* Routledge, New York.

Read, J. 1998 'Child abuse and severity of disturbance among adult psychiatric inpatients' *Child Abuse and Neglect* vol. 22, no. 5, pp. 359–68.

Real, T. 1990 'The use of self in constuctivist/systemic therapy' *Family Process* vol. 29, pp. 255–71.

Real, T. 1995 'Fathering our sons, refathering ourselves: Some thoughts on transforming legacies' *Journal of Feminist Family Therapy* vol. 7, nos. 1/2, pp. 27–44.

Reinharz, S. 1992 *Feminist Methods in Social Research* Oxford University Press, New York.

Report to National Crime Prevention 1999 *Ending Domestic Violence? Programs for Perpetrators* Commonwealth Attorney General's Department, Canberra.

Richardson D. ed. 1996 *Theorising Heterosexuality: Telling it Straight* Open University Press, Philadelphia.

Richardson D. 1996 'Heterosexuality and Social Theory' *Theorising Heterosexuality: Telling it Straight* ed. D. Richardson, Open University Press, Philadelphia.

Richmond, M. 1917 *Social Diagnosis* Russel Sage Foundation, New York.

Roberts, R. 1989a 'The influence of homophobia and heterosexism on social work education' *AASW Newsletter* vol. 3, pp. 8–9.

Roberts, R. 1989b 'Challenging heterosexist assumptions in social work education' *Advances in Social Welfare Education* eds D. James and T. Vinson, University of New South Wales, Kensington, Sydney.

Roberts, R. 1990 *Lessons for the Past: Issues for Social Work Theory* Routledge, London.

Roberts, R. 1994 'Challenging the uncritical application of HIV/AIDS politics to rural contexts' *Australian Social Work* vol. 47, no. 4, pp. 11–19.

Roberts, R. 1995 'A "fair go for all?": Discrimination and the experiences of some men who have sex with men in the bush' *Communication and Culture in Rural Areas* ed. P. Share, Charles Sturt University, Centre for Rural Social Research, Wagga Wagga.

Roberts, R. 1996 'School experiences of some rural gay men coping with "countrymindedness"' *Gay and Lesbian Perspectives III—More Essays in Australian Gay Male Culture* ed. G. Wotherspoon, Department of

Economic History and the Australian Centre for Lesbian and Gay Research, University of Sydney, Sydney.

Roberts, R. 2000 'Work with gay men and lesbians' *Fields of Social Work* eds. M. Alston and J. McKinnon, Oxford University Press, Sydney.

Rofes, E. 1996 *Reviving the Tribe: Regenerating Gay Men's Sexuality and Culture in the Ongoing Epidemic* Harrington Park Press, Binghamton.

Romano, E. and De Luca, R.V. 1997 'Exploring the relationship between childhood sexual abuse and adult sexual perpetration' *Journal of Family Violence* vol. 12, no. 1, pp. 85–97.

Rosen, L.N. and Martin, L. 1996 'Impact of childhood abuse history on psychological symptoms among male and female soldiers in the U.S. Army' *Child Abuse and Neglect* vol. 20, no. 12. pp. 1149–60.

Rosenman, S. 1998 Letter to the editor *Australasian Journal on Ageing* vol. 17, no. 3, p. 151.

Rowan, J 1997 *Healing the Male Psyche: Therapy as Initiation* Routledge, London.

Royal Commission into Aboriginal Deaths in Custody 1991 *National Report* Canberra, Australian Government Publishing Service, Canberra.

Rubinstein, R. 1996 'Is aging more problematic for women than men?' *Controversial Issues in Aging* eds A. Scharlach and L. Kaye, Allyn and Bacon, Needham Heights, MA.

Ruether, R. 1992 'Patriarchy and the men's movement: Part of the problem or part of the solution' *Women Respond to the Men's Movement* ed. K. Hagen, Harper, San Francisco.

Russell, M. 1995 *Confronting Abusive Beliefs: Group Treatment for Abusive Men* Sage, Thousand Oaks.

Ruthchild, C. 1997 'Don't frighten the horses! A systemic perspective on violence against lesbians and gay men' *Homophobic Violence* eds G. Mason & S. Tomsen, Hawkins Press, Sydney.

Ryan, G., Miyoshi, T.J., Metzner, J.L., Krugman, R.D. and Fryer, G.E. 1996 'Trends in a national sample of sexually abusive youths' *Journal of the American Academy of Child and Adolescent Psychiatry* vol. 35, no. 1, p. 17(9).

Sabo, D. and Gordon, F. 1995. 'Rethinking men's health and illness' *Men's Health and Illness: Gender, Power and the Body* eds D. Sabo and F. Gordon, Sage, Thousand Oaks.

Said, E. 1968 *Orientalism* Vintage, London.

Sampson, R. and Lamb J. 1995 *Crime in the Making* Harvard University Press, Cambridge.

Samuels, A. 1993 *The Political Psyche* Routledge, London.

Sanday, P.R. 1981 *Female Power and Male Dominance* Cambridge University Press, Cambridge.

Satariano, William A. 1997 'The physical health of older men: The signifi-cance of the social and physical environment' *Elderly Men: Special*

Problems and Professional Challenges eds J. Kosberg and L. Kaye, Springer, New York.

Sawyer, J. 1974 'On male liberation' *Men and Masculinity* eds J. Pleck & J. Sawyer, Prentice Hall, Englewood Cliffs.

Schembri, A. 1992 *Off Our Backs: A Study into Anti-lesbian Violence* Gay and Lesbian Rights Lobby of New South Wales, Sydney.

Schnarch, D. 1997 *Passionate Marriage* Norton, New York.

Schutz, A., 1972 *The Phenomenology of the Social World* Heinemann, London.

Schwalbe, M. 1993 'Why mythopoetic men don't flock to NOMAS' *Masculinities* vol. 1, nos. 3 /4, pp. 68–72.

Schwalbe, M. 1996 *Unlocking the Iron Cage* Oxford University Press.

Schwartz, A. 1974 'A transactional view of the aging process' *Professional Obligations and Approaches to the Aged* eds A. Schwartz and I. Mensh, Charles C. Thomas, Springfield, Ill.

Sedgwick, E. 1990 *Epistemology of the Closet* University of California Press, Berkeley.

Segal, L. 1987 *Is The Future Female?: Troubled Thoughts on Contemporary Feminism* Virago, London.

Seidler, V. 1989 *Rediscovering Masculinity: Reason, Language and Sexuality* Routledge, London.

Selvini-Palazzoli, M., Boscolo, L., Cecchin, G. and Prata, G. 1980 'Hypothesizing-circularity-neutrality: Three guidelines for the conductor of the session' *Family Process* vol. 19, no. 1, pp. 3–13.

Shaw, E., and Beauchamp, J. 1999 'Engaging and retaining men in therapy: Issues for female therapists working with men in relationship counselling' Paper presented at *Men in Relationships Forum* Canberra, 1998.

Shaw, E., Bouris, A., Pye, S. 1996 'The family safety model: A comprehensive strategy for working with domestic violence' *The Australian and New Zealand Journal of Family Therapy* vol. 17, no. 31, pp. 126–36.

Sidoti, C. 1999 *Issues and Strategies Around Couple Based Discrimination* Human Rights and Equal Opportunity Commission, Canberra.

Sigmon, S.T., Greene, M.P., Rohan, K.J. and Nichols, J.E. 1996 'Coping and adjustment in male and female survivors of childhood sexual abuse' *Journal of Child Sexual Abuse* vol. 5, no. 3, pp. 57–75.

Silver, E. 1991 'Should I give advice?: A systemic view' *Journal of Family Therapy* vol. 13, pp. 295–309.

Silverstein, O. and Rashbaum, B. 1994 *The Courage to Raise Good Men* Penguin, New York.

Silverstone, B. and Burack-Weiss, A. 1983 *Social Work Practice with the Elderly and their Families* Charles C. Thomas, Springfield, Ill.

Sim, J. 1994 'Tougher than the rest? Men in prison' *Just Boys Doing Business? Men, Masculinities and Crime* eds T. Newburn & E. Stanko, Routledge, London.

Skuse, D., Bentovim, A., Hodges, J., Stevenson, J., Andreou, C., Lanyado, M., New, M., Williams, B. and McMillan, D. 1998 'Risk factors for the development of sexually abusive behaviour in sexually victimised adolescent boys: cross sectional study' *British Medical Journal* vol. 317, no. 7052, p. 175(5).

Smith, D. and Stewart J. 1997 'Probation and Social Exclusion' *Social Policy and Administration* vol. 31, no. 5, pp. 96–115.

Smith, G. 1996 'Dichotomies in the making of men' *Men's Ways of Being* eds C. McLean, M. Carey & C. White. Westview Press, Boulder, Colorado.

Solomon, K. and Szwabo, P. 1994 'The work-oriented culture: Success and power in elderly men' *Older Men's Lives* ed. E. Thompson Jr., Sage, Thousand Oaks, CA.

South Australian Health Commission 1997 *The South Australian Men's Health Policy Background Paper* Adelaide.

Spock, J. Blashfield, R. and Smith, B. 1990 'Gender weighting of DSM-IIIR personality disorder criteria' *American Journal of Psychiatry* no. 147, pp. 586–90.

Stanko, E. 1994 'Challenging the problem of men's individual violence' *Just Boys Doing Business? Men, Masculinities and Crime* eds T. Newburn & E. Stanko, Routledge, London.

Stanley, J. and Goddard, C. 1993 'The association between child abuse and other family violence' *Australian Social Work* vol. 46, no. 2, pp. 3–8.

Steiner, C. 1986 *When a Man Loves a Woman: Sexual and Emotional Literacy for the Modern Man* Grove Press, New York.

Sterba, J. 1998 'Is feminism good for men and are men good for feminism?' *Men Doing Feminism* ed. T. Digby, Routledge, London.

Stern, D. 1985 *The Interpersonal World of the Infant* Basic Books, New York.

Suicide Prevention Task Force 1997 *Suicide Prevention: Victorian Task Force Report* Victorian Government, Melbourne.

Swan, P. and Raphael, B. 1996 *Ways Forward* National Consultancy Report on Aboriginal and Torres Strait Islander Mental Health, Australian Government Publishing Service, Canberra.

Swift, M.B. 1998 *Male Sexual Victimisation: The Silenced Victims* Masters Thesis, RMIT University, Melbourne.

Swigonski, M. 1993 'Feminist standpoint theory and the question of social work research' *Affilia* vol. 8, no. 2, pp. 171–83.

Taggart, N. 1992 'Book review: Men in therapy; The challenge of change' by R. Myth and R. Pasick, *Journal of Feminist Family Therapy* vol. 4, no. 1, pp. 96–8.

Tamasese, K. and Waldegrave, C. 1993 'Cultural and gender accountability in the "Just Therapy" approach' *Journal of Feminist Family Therapy* vol. 5, no. 2, pp. 29–45.

Tamasese, K. and Walgrave, C. 1994 'Cultural and gender accountability in the "Just Therapy" approach' *Dulwich Centre Newsletter* Dulwich Centre Publications, Adelaide, no. 2 & 3, pp. 55–67.

Tarmas, R. 1996 *The Passion of the Western Mind* Pimlico, London.

Taubman, S. 1986 'Beyond the bravado: Sex roles and the exploitative male' *Social Work* vol. 31, no. 1, pp. 12–18.

Taylor, J. 1990 *Giving Women Voice: Feminism and Women's Services* Brotherhood of St. Laurence, Melbourne.

Thomas, D. *Not Guilty: In Defence of the Modern Man.* Weidenfeld and Nicholson, London.

Thompson, D. 1985 *Flaws in the Social Fabric: Homosexuals and Society in Sydney* George Allen & Unwin, Sydney.

Thompson Jnr. E. ed. 1994 *Older Men's Lives* Sage, Thousand Oaks, CA.

Thompson, Jnr. E. 1994 'Older men as invisible men in contemporary society' *Older Men's Lives* ed. E. Thompson, Sage, Thousand Oaks, CA.

Thompson, N. 1995 'Men and anti-sexism' *British Journal of Social Work* vol. 25, no. 4, pp. 459–75.

Thompson, N. 1998 *Promoting Equality: Challenging Discrimination and Oppression in the Human Services* Macmillan, London.

Thorne-Finch, R. 1992 *Ending The Silence: The Origins and Treatment of Male Violence Against Women* University of Toronto Press, Toronto.

Trotter, C. 1999 *Working with Involuntary Clients: A Guide to Practice* Allen & Unwin, Sydney.

Trudinger, M., Boyd, C. and Melrose, P. 1998 'Questioning sexuality: A workshop in progress' *Dulwich Centre Journal* Dulwich Centre Publications, Adelaide, no. 4, pp. 9–16.

Turk, S., Rose, T. and Gatz, M. 1996 'The significance of gender in the treatment of older adults' *The Practical Handbook of Clinical Gerontology* eds L. Carstensen, B. Edelstern & L. Dornbrand, Sage, Thousand Oaks, CA.

Ungerson, C. 1983 'Why do women care' *A labour of love: Women, work and caring* eds J. Finch & D. Groves, Routledge and Kegan Paul, London.

Vaillant, G. 1994 '"Successful aging" and psychosocial well-being: Evidence from a 45 year study' *Older Men's Lives* ed. E. Thompson Jr., Sage, Thousand Oaks, CA.

Victorian Taskforce Report, 1997 *Suicide Prevention* Australian Government Publishing Service, Canberra.

Wadham, B. 1997 'The new men's health: A media marvel' *Social Alternatives* vol. 16, no. 3, pp. 19–22.

Walker, A. 1980 'The social creation of poverty and dependency in old age' *Journal of Social Policy* vol. 9, no. 1, pp. 49–75.

Walton, R. 1975 *Women in Social Work* Routledge & Kegan Paul, London.

Weeks, W. 1994 *Women Working Together: Lessons From Feminist Women's Services* Longman Cheshire, Melbourne.

Weingarten K. 1991 'The discourses of intimacy: Adding a social constructionist and feminist view' *Family Process* vol. 30, no. 3, pp. 285–306.

White, C. ed. 1995 'Discussions, dialogues and interviews about homophobia and heterosexual dominance' *Comment* no. 2, Dulwich Centre Publications, Adelaide.

White, M. 1992 *Experience, Narrative and Imagination* Dulwich Centre Publications, Adelaide.

White, M. and Epstein, D. 1989 *Literate Means to Therapeutic Ends* Dulwich Centre Publications, Adelaide.

White, Phillip 1999 *The Prison Population in 1998: A Statistical Review* Research Findings No. 94, Home Office Research, Development and Statistics Directorate, London.

Widigier, T. and Weissman, M. 1991 'Epidemiology of borderline personality disorder' *Hospital and Community Psychiatry* vol. 42, pp. 1015–19.

Williams. C. 1996 *Fathers and Sons* Angus and Robertson, Sydney.

Williams C. and Thorpe, B. 1992 *Beyond Industrial Sociology: The Work of Men and Women* Allen & Unwin, Sydney.

Wilson, E. 1983 *What is to be done about violence against women?* Penguin, London.

Wolf-Light, P. 1999 'Men, violence and love' *Working with Men for Change* ed. J. Wild, UCL Press, London.

Women's Information Switchboard 1980 *Phone In* Women's Information Switchboard, Adelaide.

Wotherspoon, G. 1991 *City of the Plain: History of a Gay Sub-Culture* Hale & Iremonger, Sydney.

Young, J., Perlesz, A., Paterson, R., O'Hanlon, B., Newbold, A., Chaplin, R. & Bridge, S. 1989 'The reflecting team process in training' *Australian and New Zealand Journal of Family Therapy* vol. 10, no. 2, pp. 69–74.

Index

For Product Safety Concerns and Information please contact our EU
representative GPSR@taylorandfrancis.com
Taylor & Francis Verlag GmbH, Kaufingerstraße 24, 80331 München, Germany

www.ingramcontent.com/pod-product-compliance
Lightning Source LLC
Chambersburg PA
CBHW071416290326
41932CB00046B/1890